DATE DUE

With the assistance of

RICHARD DRUSS, M.D.
Assistant Professor of Clinical Psychiatry,
Columbia University, College of Physicians and Surgeons

JOSEPH SWEETING, M.D.
Associate Professor of Clinical Medicine,
Columbia University, College of Physicians and Surgeons

1977
W. B. SAUNDERS COMPANY
Philadelphia • London • Toronto

PSYCHOTHERAPY in CHRONIC ULCERATIVE COLITIS

AARON KARUSH, M.D.
Professor of Clinical Psychiatry, Columbia University,
College of Physicians and Surgeons

and

GEORGE E. DANIELS, M.D.
Former Clinical Professor of Psychiatry, Columbia University,
College of Physicians and Surgeons

CHARLES FLOOD, M.D.
Professor of Clinical Medicine Emeritus, Columbia University,
College of Physicians and Surgeons

JOHN F. O'CONNOR, M.D.
Associate Clinical Professor of Psychiatry,
Columbia University, College of Physicians and Surgeons

W. B. Saunders Company: West Washington Square
Philadelphia, PA 19105

1 St. Anne's Road
Eastbourne, East Sussex BN21 3UN, England

1 Goldthorne Avenue
Toronto, Ontario M8Z 5T9, Canada

Library of Congress Cataloging in Publication Data

Karush, Aaron.

Psychotherapy in chronic ulcerative colitis.

Includes index.

1. Ulcerative colitis—Psychosomatic aspects. 2. Psychotherapy. I. Title. [DNLM: 1. Colitis, Ulcerative—Therapy. 2. Psychotherapy. WI522 P974]

RC862.U5K37 616.3′44 76–28939

ISBN 0–7216–5293–X

Psychotherapy in Chronic Ulcerative Colitis ISBN 0-7216-5293-X

Last digit is the print number: 8 7 6 5 4 3 2 1

PREFACE

For some 40 years, there has been a combined effort by internists, psychiatrists and surgeons at the Columbia–Presbyterian Medical Center in New York to clarify the complex course and nature of chronic ulcerative colitis. The group has recognized that the disease process reflected the possible convergence of many factors—genetic, constitutional, infectious and psychological, to name but a few. In order to evaluate changing therapeutic approaches, it was agreed that long-term follow-up studies were essential.

As time went on, therapies changed. Sulfonamides administered internally or topically were largely replaced, with the exception of Azulfidine, by steroids, radical surgery and psychotherapy. The changing fashions in treatment testify to the continuing challenge this destructive illness still presents.

Although we still do not have a full understanding of the multifaceted cause of ulcerative colitis, significant data have been gathered that have helped us to make better order of our findings and the sometimes contradictory observations of others.

The purpose of this book is to clarify the natural progression of the disease and to indicate the kind of psychotherapy that may best help to alleviate the pathological process itself or at least improve the general functioning of the patient. In addition, the role of psychological factors in the predisposition to the illness and their impact upon the outcome of combined medical and psychiatric treatment is discussed at some length.

As we show, the value of psychotherapy is not invariable. It cannot help every patient. In the succeeding chapters, the basis for selecting those patients who might reasonably be expected to benefit from the addition of psychotherapy and the criteria for choosing the kind of psychotherapeutic approach best suited to a particular patient are documented.

Our discussion is directed primarily toward psychotherapists, most of whom will be psychiatrists. It is hoped, however, that internists who are responsible for planning the treatment of patients with colitis will find our suggestions useful to themselves, as well. There will always be a sizable proportion of patients whose life situations and general adjustment can be immediately helped by the internist himself. It is toward this group of patients and physicians as well as toward specially trained psychotherapists that our findings and hypotheses about predisposition and intervention are directed.

THE AUTHORS

ACKNOWLEDGMENTS

The authors owe far more, individually and collectively, than can be adequately acknowledged to the many colleagues and coworkers whose dedicated participation and cooperation helped us to complete the various studies that have made this book possible. We are especially indebted to the faculty and postgraduate students of the Columbia Psychoanalytic Clinic for Training and Research, who treated many of our patients.

There are several colleagues, however, whom we wish to single out for their personal interest or for their invaluable contributions to our work. Dr. Agnes Conrad of the Presbyterian Hospital in New York and Dr. Walter L. Palmer of Chicago were among the first to give encouragement to Dr. George Daniels during his early investigations. In later years, Dr. Michael J. Lepore of the Department of Medicine, Dr. Robert B. Hiatt and Dr. John Prudden, both of the Department of Surgery, Dr. Leon Moses (deceased) and Mrs. Leonore Stern actively took part in various aspects of our studies at the Columbia–Presbyterian Medical Center, and we express our deepest gratitude to them. Dr. Robert Weiss and Dr. Robert Senescu were particularly helpful during our follow-up investigations, and we are grateful to John W. Fertig, Professor Emeritus of Biostatistics, and to Mrs. Livia R. Turgeon, Research Associate, for advice and guidance in the organization of the statistical data.

To Dr. Lawrence C. Kolb, former Chairman of the Department of Psychiatry at Columbia University and presently Commissioner of Mental Hygiene in New York State, we are especially indebted for his unflagging interest and for his encouragement to organize our findings and hypotheses for this publication.

Finally, and most important, we thank our patients, whose courage despite much suffering sustained our efforts to find a deeper understanding of their illness and more effective ways to undo its unhappy effects upon their lives.

CONTENTS

Chapter One

THE GENERAL COURSE OF CHRONIC ULCERATIVE COLITIS

The clinical course of nonspecific ulcerative colitis is generally characterized by periods of active symptoms that alternate with periods of freedom from symptoms. The quiescent periods, or remissions, tend to last longer than the periods of exacerbation, but the duration of both varies greatly. Some patients experience periods of active disease that last for years. Remission may nevertheless occasionally occur after a year or more of active symptoms and may continue for long periods of time. In more than half the patients with ulcerative colitis, one can anticipate that symptomatic remission will take place within six months. The remission will usually, however, be followed by a relapse after a period of time.

During the last 20 years, most patients with ulcerative colitis have received treatment with steroids or Azulfidine (salicylazosulfapyridine), drugs that are effective in controlling symptoms in many patients. Prior to 1950, ulcerative colitis was treated with a variety of other medications that in retrospect probably had only a slight effect on the course of the disease. The agents that were used during the earlier years included antispasmodics, the belladonna series, the synthetic quaternary ammonium compounds, sedatives such as barbiturates, antimicrobial agents such as the absorbable and non-absorbable sulfonamide compounds, and various antibiotics including penicillin, the tetracyclines and chloramphenicol.

The clinical picture of ulcerative colitis seen prior to 1950 may be regarded as representative of the natural history of the disease, somewhat modified by therapeutic procedures. During these earlier years, numerous studies reported that about two thirds of symptomatic patients with ulcerative colitis improved on a variety of treatments employed during a limited period of study. Short-term improvement was observed in about 60 to 80 per cent of patients treated with sulfonamide drugs, various antibiotics and other types of supportive therapy.[1-10]

The present account portrays the clinical course of the disease as seen in our Ulcerative Colitis Clinic prior to the introduction of steroids.

The impact of steroid and Azulfidine therapy is then reviewed. An attempt is also made to reclassify the patients under follow-up study into two categories—those with typical ulcerative colitis and those with Crohn's disease of the large bowel ("atypical colitis")—in order to evaluate retrospectively the prognostic significance of such classifications.

The course of ulcerative colitis may conveniently be represented in terms of periods of exacerbation ("attacks") and periods of remission (Fig. 1–1). An attack is defined as the occurrence of diarrhea for a minimum of one week or as the presence of any rectal bleeding. Diarrhea or bleeding almost always occurs during any clinical exacerbation of ulcerative colitis. Other symptoms such as abdominal pain, joint pains or fever may also be present but are less frequent and are not useful as continuous parameters of the clinical activity of the disease.

Remission is also defined in symptomatic terms. We have arbitrarily considered the absence of symptoms and the presence of formed stools containing no blood for a minimum of one month to be a symptomatic remission. Shorter periods of freedom from symptoms are not designated as remissions.

Attacks may be analyzed in terms of severity as well as duration. The extent of the disturbance in bowel function is again the most sensitive measure of the activity of the inflammatory process. The amount of diarrhea increases with the severity of the total clinical picture. We have assigned numerical values for severity in ascending order according to the severity of the symptoms. This is a reversal of the system used in prior publications.[10]

0. Formed stools without blood.
1. Loose stools numbering up to five per day.
2. Moderate symptoms with 6 to 10 stools daily; the patient is ambulatory.
3. Incapacitating symptoms, usually requiring hospitalization.

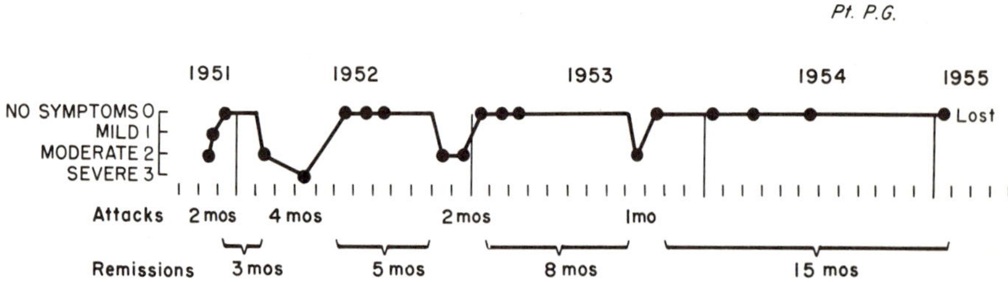

Figure 1–1 Graph of the clinical course of a patient with ulcerative colitis, demonstrating the duration and the severity of each attack and the duration of each remission. This method was used to derive the data shown in the tables.

CLINICAL COURSE UNDER PRESTEROID MEDICAL SUPPORTIVE THERAPY

The long-term behavior of ulcerative colitis before steroids came into general use was recorded by this Clinic in 1956 for a series of patients who had been under continuous observation.[10] The present report amplifies the description that was published previously. The group of patients considered here did not receive steroids, Azulfidine or any formal program of psychotherapy during the period under consideration. This experience is presented, therefore, as being representative of the natural history of ulcerative colitis insofar as practicable.

This series consisted of 103 patients with evidence of inflammatory disease of the large bowel, manifested in all instances on sigmoidoscopic examination and, in most, on roentgenographic examination as well. The diagnostic criteria were those that had been generally accepted for such a diagnosis prior to 1960. Some of the patients were undoubtedly suffering from granulomatous colitis; this is later discussed in detail.

All patients were more than 14 years of age, with an average age of 35 years. There were 50 males and 53 females; 5 patients were black. Forty patients were Jewish, and 36 were Catholics. At the time of the first referred attack, 20 patients had only proctitis with no evidence of colonic involvement on x-ray examination. Sixty-three had partial colonic involvement on x-ray examination, and 20 had universal involvement of the colon and the rectum. Only 3 patients had x-ray evidence of ileal involvement when initially seen.

The clinical course of this series of patients through the first three attacks and the first three periods of remission after referral to our Clinic is summarized in Table 1–1. During these three attacks, 14 patients (14 per cent) went to surgery. Thirty-three patients were lost to follow-up while still having active symptoms. Most of the latter were individuals with intractable symptoms who had been under treatment many months before disappearing from follow-up. One death occurred after conservative therapy, and four deaths occurred postoperatively—a mortality rate of 5 per cent.

The average duration of the first three attacks ranged from 4.3 to 4.8 months (Fig. 1–2) and was remarkably uniform. No essential difference in duration was noted between the first, the second and the third attacks. On the other hand, there was a wide variation in the duration of attacks for individual patients, ranging from 1 to more than 30 months.

The average duration of remissions ranged from 14 to 18 months. Again, little difference was noted in the average duration of the remissions between the first and second and between the second and third attacks. In other words, it appears that the duration of a remission is independent of the number of previous attacks. Individual remissions varied

TABLE 1–1 Results of Medical Supportive (Presteroid) Therapy in Ulcerative Colitis

FIRST REFERRED ATTACK					REMITTERS AFTER FIRST ATTACK		
Outcome of Attack	**No. of Patients**	**Average Severity**	**Average Duration** *(months)*	**Deaths**	**Outcome for Remitters**	**No. of Patients**	**Average Duration** *(months)*
Operations	11	3.0	12.2[a]	3	Still in remission	2	174.0[c]
Lost before remission	16	2.7	12.7[a]	1	Lost in remission	12	32.3[a]
Data incomplete	3				Data incomplete	3	
Went into remission	73	2.3	4.8[b]		Followed to next attack	59	15.4[d]
Total	103			4	Total	76[e]	

SECOND ATTACK					REMITTERS AFTER SECOND ATTACK		
Outcome of Attack	**No. of Patients**	**Average Severity**	**Average Duration** *(months)*	**Deaths**	**Outcome for Remitters**	**No. of Patients**	**Average Duration** *(months)*
Operations	1	3.0	1.0	1	Still in remission	1	150.0[c]
Lost before remission	11	2.0	10.2[a]		Lost in remission	7	19.0[a]
Data incomplete	3				Data incomplete	2	
Went into remission	47	1.6	4.7[f]		Followed to next attack	40	14.0[g]
Total	62			1	Total	50	

	THIRD ATTACK				REMITTERS AFTER THIRD ATTACK		
Outcome of Attack	No. of Patients	Average Severity	Average Duration (*months*)	Deaths	Outcome for Remitters	No. of Patients	Average Duration (*months*)
Operations	2	3.0	2.5[a]		Still in remission	0	
Lost before remission	6	2.0	1.0[a]		Lost in remission	4	50.0[a]
Data incomplete	2				Data incomplete	1	
Went into remission	32	1.4	4.3[h]		Followed to next attack	29	18.0[i]
Total	42				Total	34	

This table summarizes the outcomes for 103 patients followed continuously who were on supportive treatment without steroids, Azulfidine or formal psychotherapy.

[a]Duration to loss or surgery.

[b]Range – 1 to 36 months.

[c]Up to the present.

[d]Range – 1 to 120 months.

[e]These 76 patients comprise the 73 individuals who went into remission during the first attack, plus the 3 patients who were seen in the first attack whose data were incomplete for that attack. This system of classification applies also to the subsequent tabulations.

[f]Range – 1 to 30 months.

[g]Range – 3 to 180 months.

[h]Range – 1 to 24 months.

[i]Range – 1 to 180 months.

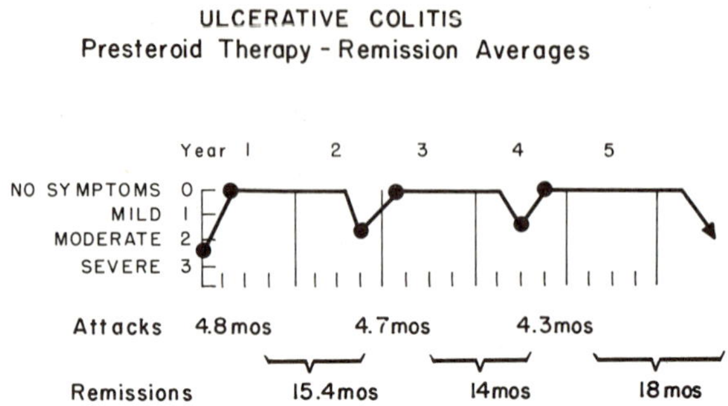

Figure 1–2 Graph of the average clinical course of ulcerative colitis under presteroid supportive therapy. The averages are derived from records of 103 patients and from the data in Table 1–1.

widely, lasting from 1 month to more than 10 years. About one third of all remissions lasted more than a year.

REMISSION AND RELAPSE RATE

The short-term prognosis for ulcerative colitis may also be expressed in terms of the proportion of patients who experience remission within a set period of time. The percentage of patients who enter a remission in the course of a six-month period serves as a useful guide in the management of individual patients. It must be noted, however, that this method of tabulation fails to record a number of important details about the treatment failures, such as losses to follow-up and deaths, and does not reflect the most serious aspects of the picture.

The average six-month remission rate for the 103 patients for all three attacks was 57 per cent (Table 1–2). No significant difference in the rate of remission was seen during the first, the second and the third

TABLE 1–2 Medical Supportive Therapy (Presteroid)

	NO. OF EPISODES	NO. GOING INTO REMISSION EACH MONTH* 1 mo.	2 mos.	3 mos.	4 mos.	5 mos.	6 mos.	REMISSION RATE
First referred attack	103	17	14	9	7	3	4	54 (52%)
Second referred attack	62	13	9	8	4	3	1	38 (61%)
Third referred attack	42	12	7	1	2	1	3	26 (62%)
Totals	207	42	30	18	13	7	8	118 (57%)

*Monthly incidence of symptomatic remissions in 103 patients on supportive therapy (without steroids, Azulfidine or psychotherapy). The remission rate was a little lower for the first referred attack, but the differences are small.

TABLE 1–3 Medical Supportive Therapy (Presteroid)

	NO. OF EPISODES	NO. GOING INTO RELAPSE EACH MONTH* 1 mo.	2 mos.	3 mos.	4 mos.	5 mos.	6 mos.	RELAPSE TOTAL
First remission	76	1	9	6	3	4	4	27 (36%)
Second remission	50	1	2	1	2	4	7	17 (34%)
Third remission	34	0	0	4	3	2	2	11 (33%)
Totals	160	2	11	11	8	10	13	55 (34%)

*Monthly incidence of relapses in 103 patients after supportive therapy (no steroids, Azulfidine or psychotherapy). The frequency of relapse was the same in the first, the second and the third remissions.

referred attacks. The rate for each of these attacks varied from 52 to 62 per cent. Following symptomatic remission, 34 per cent of patients relapsed within six months (Table 1–3). The frequency of relapses was roughly the same after the first, the second and the third attacks. The relapse rate remained remarkably constant for each observed period of remission.

Although there was little variation in the duration of remissions and in the number of relapses during the course of the disease, there was a marked difference between the severity of the first referred attack and the severity of subsequent attacks in this series. The first referred attack was usually more severe than the subsequent ones and was commonly incapacitating (see Table 1–1). Most of the operations in the group were done at the time of the first referred attack; 10 per cent of patients underwent surgery then. For another 20 per cent of patients having their first attack, surgery was often considered because of the severity of the illness. The largest percentage of patients lost to follow-up were lost during their first referred attack. As stated earlier, these were often individuals who continued to have severe and protracted symptoms during follow-up. It may be that the severity of the first referred attack in this series should be attributed to the tendency of patients with severe and frustrating symptoms to seek advice in university centers and large private clinics. Most of the second and third attacks observed in this series were mild or moderate.

Effect of Steroid Therapy

The development of steroids in 1950 resulted in a major change in the management of ulcerative colitis. In the course of a few years, a British cooperative controlled study as well as many other investigations demonstrated convincingly that steroids in moderate dosage will induce a symptomatic remission in many patients with ulcerative colitis.[11, 12] Subsequent experience continues to confirm this.

TABLE 1–4 Medical Supportive Therapy and Steroid Therapy Symptomatic Remission Rates*

TYPE OF THERAPY	NO. OF EPISODES	NO. ENTERING REMISSION EACH MONTH 1 mo.	2 mos.	3 mos.	4 mos.	5 mos.	6 mos.	REMISSION TOTAL
Presteroid	272	55	38	39	14	10	12	168 (60%)
Steroid	101	45	14	5	5	1	5	75 (75%)

*Remission rates of patients treated with supportive therapy compared with incidence of remissions of those given steroids. All patients had inflammatory disease of the colon without small bowel involvement.

Our own experience with steroids can conveniently be expressed in terms of remission and relapse rates.[13] A symptomatic remission takes place within one month in about half the patients treated with steroids (Table 1–4). Although steroids accelerate remission, it is also noteworthy that the cumulative six-month remission rate resulting from steroid therapy is not very different from that observed in follow-up studies of patients prior to the introduction of steroids. In this study, 75 per cent of steroid-treated patients entered remission within six months, as compared with 60 per cent during the presteroid era.

It appears that there is a penalty for the early remission induced by steroids, however. Our figures indicate that there is an increased tendency to relapse as the drug is withdrawn. The six-month relapse rate in steroid-treated patients in the series was 53 per cent. In the presteroid period, the six-month relapse rate was only 33 per cent. As shown in Table 1–5, more than half the relapses in the steroid-treated patients were incident to tapering off or stopping steroids (Table 1–5). This is presumably because the usual practice in steroid administration had been to begin to taper the dosage shortly after remission had taken place. Steroids have commonly been tapered off or discontinued within two to three months after the onset of steroid therapy. Whereas steroids may rapidly induce a remission, the patient may be more apt to have an early recurrence of symptoms as the steroids are withdrawn.

TABLE 1–5 Medical Supportive Therapy and Steroid Therapy Symptomatic Relapse Rates

TYPE OF THERAPY	NO. OF EPISODES	NO. OF RELAPSES EACH MONTH 1 to 2 mos.	3 to 6 mos.	TOTAL IN 6 MOS.	PER CENT OF RELAPSES IN 6 MOS.
Presteroid	101	7	26	33	33%
Steroid	90	17 (15*)	31 (16*)	48 (31*)	53%

*No. of relapses incident to tapering or stopping steroid therapy. Note the large proportion of relapses that occurred within two months after steroid dosage was tapered off.

Effect of Azulfidine Therapy

Azulfidine (salicylazosulfapyridine) was introduced by Svartz in the treatment of ulcerative colitis in 1940. Numerous studies appear to indicate that this drug induces a symptomatic remission in many patients.[14-20]

In our experience, patients treated with Azulfidine enter remission slowly. About two months are required for 50 per cent of patients treated with this agent to achieve a symptomatic remission. It appears that patients treated with Azulfidine do not respond as rapidly as patients who receive steroids. While the British controlled studies seem to indicate that this drug is an effective one, its effect is not as dramatic as that of steroids. The value of Azulfidine in preventing relapses is currently under investigation.

REMOTE RESULTS OF MEDICAL TREATMENT

Remission and relapse rates are useful in the management of the individual with ulcerative colitis. On the other hand, the long-term outlook must be expressed by other methods of analysis. For example, it may be expressed in terms of satisfactory and unsatisfactory years of patient observation. A number of reports have indicated that approximately 50 per cent of follow-up patient years in the course of ulcerative colitis are relatively satisfactory.

Tabulation of the results by years in our series of 103 patients treated during the presteroid period gives a relatively optimistic picture (Fig. 1–3). One third of patient years were asymptomatic. Only 40 per cent of patient years were classified as containing periods of moderate or

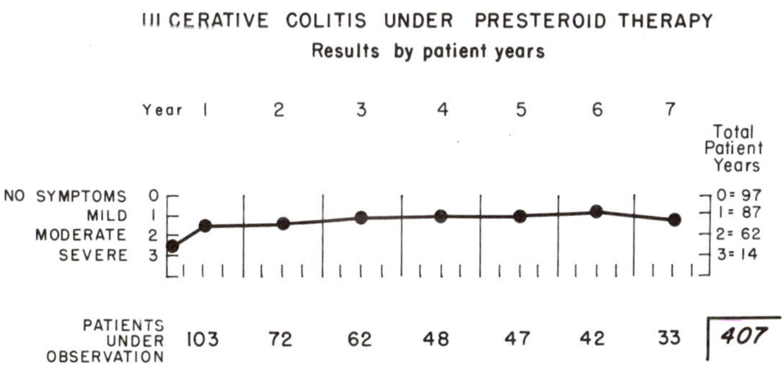

Figure 1–3 Graph of the severity of symptoms in ulcerative colitis, year by year. Each point on the curve is the average of all of the original 103 patients who remained under conservative observation each year. The maximal severity of symptoms for each patient was used to calculate these averages.

severe symptoms. One may therefore generalize that the average patient may expect symptoms to remain mild from year to year.[10, 21] This rosy outlook, however, is partly the result of the early subtraction of the more severely ill patients from the follow-up group as a result of surgical intervention or loss from follow-up.

The long-term follow-up of ulcerative colitis may also be expressed in terms of mortality tables. The data obtained in our Follow-up Clinic do not permit such a compilation. It can be noted, however, that the seven-year mortality rate for patients remaining under conservative treatment was 5 per cent. Only one of the 103 patients developed carcinoma of the large bowel. Too many patients were lost to follow-up to permit the compilation of life expectancy tables.

There are in the literature a number of interval follow-up surveys of groups of individuals shown to have ulcerative colitis.[22-26] Such data demonstrate a comparatively high cumulative mortality rate for ulcerative colitis over the years. Moreover, the measurement of cumulative death rates for large groups is very useful, as pointed out by Riis, in the evaluation of the remote effects of major therapeutic modalities, particularly surgical intervention.[26]

Edwards and Truelove reported a 10-year mortality rate of 22.6 per cent for all observed cases of ulcerative colitis.[23] They have also shown, however, that there has been a notable reduction in mortality in recent years that seems attributable in part to the use of steroids. Riis also points out that the more aggressive use of surgery is increasing the life expectancy of patients with ulcerative colitis.

ENDOSCOPIC CHANGES IN ULCERATIVE COLITIS

Sigmoidoscopic examination of most patients with active nonspecific ulcerative colitis reveals a characteristic change in the appearance of the rectal mucosa. During an acute attack, the rectal mucosa is friable, edematous and often covered with a white exudate. After symptoms subside, a gradual improvement in the proctoscopic picture takes place. The proctoscopic changes fit roughly into various stages, which may be classified as follows.[10, 27, 28]

Grade 3. A bleeding, friable, edematous mucosa often covered with exudate. This is the usual finding in the sicker patient (Color plate, Fig. 1).

Grade 2. A granular mucosa without friability or exudate. This appearance is often seen as the patient improves symptomatically (Color plate, Fig. 2).

Grade 1. Restitution of the mucosa to near normal. The mucosa remains inflamed in some areas (Color plate, Fig. 3).

Grade 0. Restitution of the mucosa to a state that usually would

TABLE 1-6 Complete Remission (Both Symptomatic and Proctoscopic)*

THERAPY	NO. OF EPISODES	1 mo.	2 mos.	3 mos.	4 mos.	5 mos.	6 mos.	REMISSION TOTAL
		NO. ENTERING FULL REMISSION EACH MONTH						
Steroids	73	10	8	6	5	1	3	33 (45%)
Azulfidine	59	7	7	5	3	1	3	26 (44%)
Presteroid	88	3	12	7	4	1	4	31 (35%)

*Complete remission frequently occurs more rapidly with steroid therapy. At six months, this advantage is less evident. (From Modern Gastroenterology. Gregor, O., and Riedl, O., eds. F. K. Schattauer, Stuttgart, 1969, p. 1006.)

not permit a diagnosis of ulcerative colitis. Loss of vascular pattern may still be noted, however. Residuals of ulcerative colitis, such as pseudopolyps, atrophy or pitting of the mucosa, may still be seen in some cases (Color plate, Figs. 4 and 5).

A complete remission of symptoms and an improvement in proctoscopic findings occur in about 40 per cent of patients within six months after the onset of treatment.[13] With steroid therapy, such a full remission takes place somewhat more rapidly than with supportive therapy or Azulfidine (Table 1-6). Symptoms disappear long before the anatomical remission occurs. Diarrhea and bleeding usually clear up weeks or months before there is a restitution of the mucosa to a normal appearance (Color plate, Figs. 4 and 5).

Serial proctoscopic examinations are also useful prognostically in ulcerative colitis (Table 1-7). It appears that the outlook for patients who achieve a full remission with restitution of the proctoscopic picture to almost normal is better than for those who achieve symptomatic remission but still have proctoscopic evidence of inflammation. The six-month relapse rate following complete remission was also substantially less than after symptomatic remission (Figs. 1-4 and 1-5).

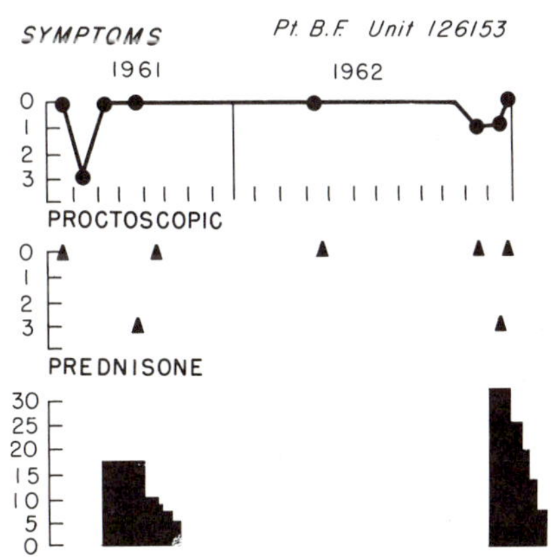

Figure 1-4 Graph of symptomatic and proctoscopic course of a patient receiving intermittent steroid therapy. Complete remission, verified by proctoscopic examination, occurred on two occasions with prednisone, in initial doses of 15 mg. and 30 mg. (shown in scale at the left). Reversion of the proctoscopic picture to normal is a favorable prognostic sign.

Figure 1 Bleeding, friable mucosa of active ulcerative colitis. This stage of inflammation is designated Grade 3.

Figure 2 Granular mucosa without friability. This picture is often seen as patient with ulcerative colitis improves. This is designated Grade 2.

Figure 3 Type of borderline changes often seen after patient has entered symptomatic remission. This is designated Grade 1.

Figure 4 No active inflammatory changes are seen in this patient with ulcerative colitis. This is designated Grade 0.

Figure 5 Patient with segmental colitis. Discrete ulceration is seen by coloscopy.

Figure 6 Patient who formerly had right-sided colitis (classified as atypical colitis). There are now diffuse changes in the rectum indistinguishable from nonspecific ulcerative colitis.

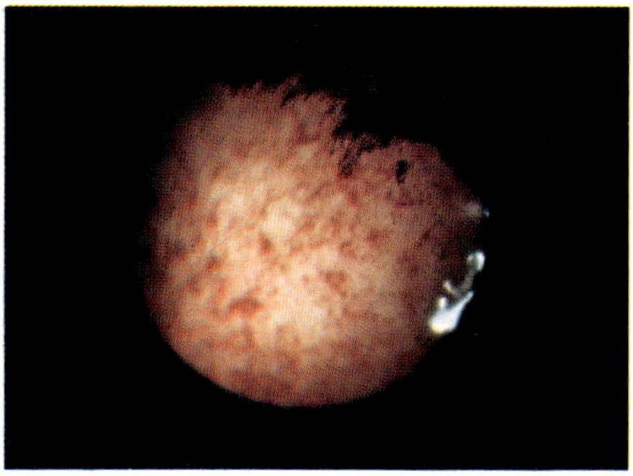

1

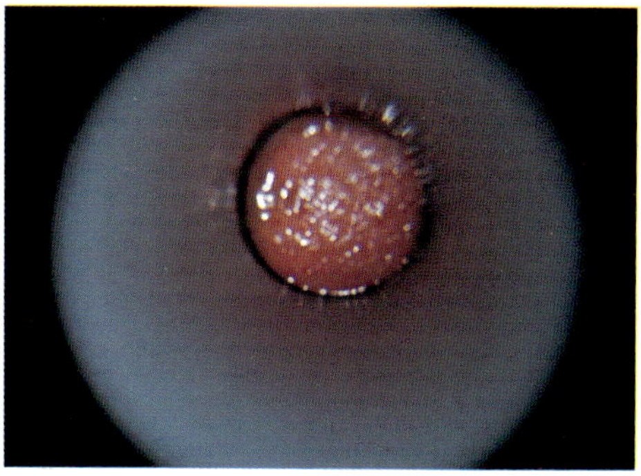

2

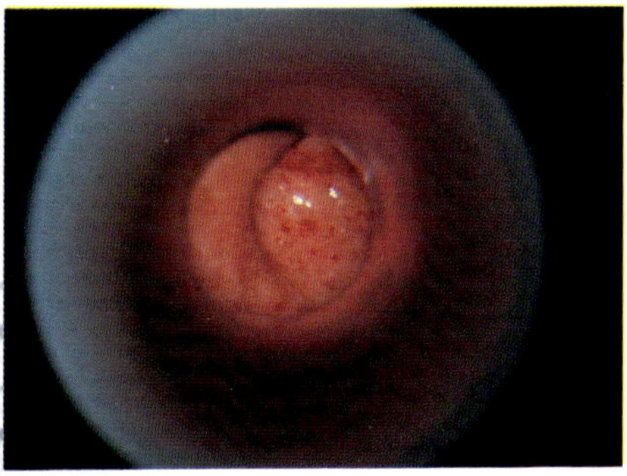

3

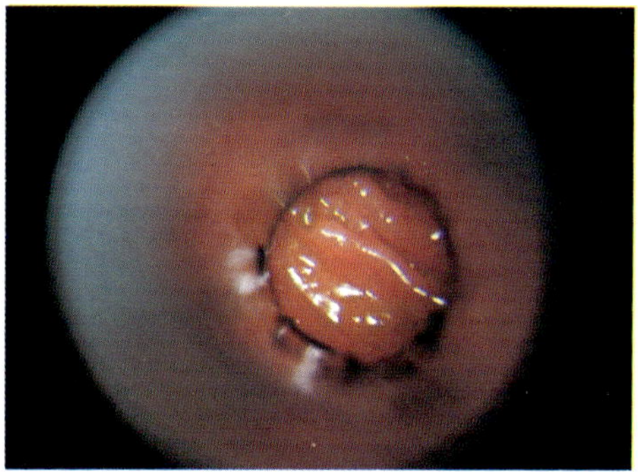

4

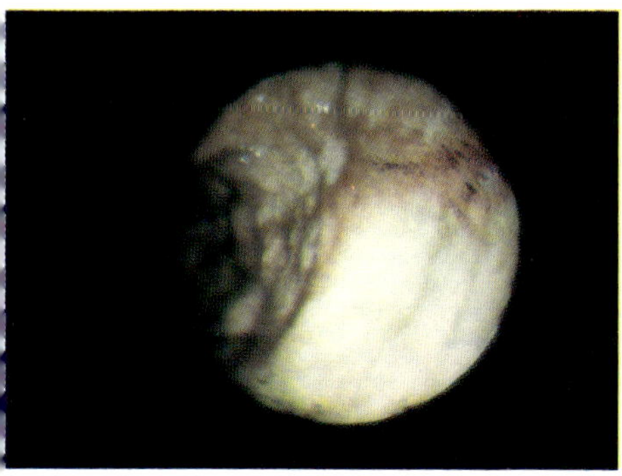

5

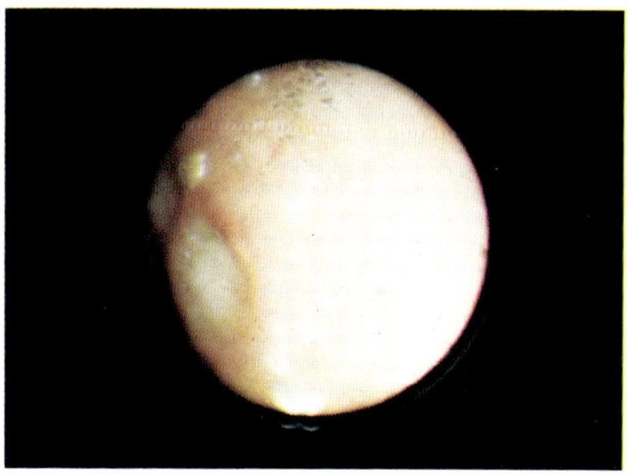

6

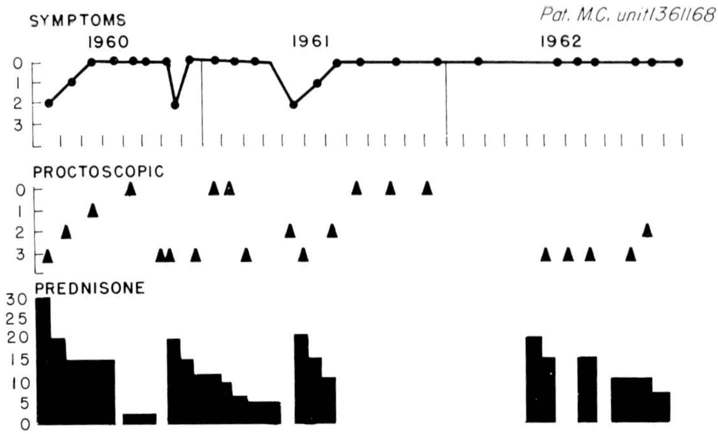

Figure 1–5 Graph of symptomatic and proctoscopic course of a patient receiving intermittent steroid therapy. The first two relapses seemed to occur after the dosage of prednisone had been decreased, as indicated on the milligram scale at the left. It is of interest that the patient was found to have had a flare-up in 1962 that was asymptomatic on proctoscopic examination. In general, proctoscopic examination is more sensitive than the symptomatic picture as a parameter of disease activity.

COLOSCOPY

The introduction of coloscopy has provided an additional method of examination of the colon in ulcerative colitis. The use of this procedure is currently recommended for patients whose symptoms are mild or absent; its use is not advised for patients with acute symptoms. Coloscopy is useful for estimating the extent of colonic involvement in patients with few or no radiological changes.

The gross picture at coloscopy in atypical granulomatous colitis is different at times from that characteristic of ulcerative colitis; one may find patchy inflammatory changes with intervening areas of relatively

TABLE 1–7 Relapse Rate Following Full Remission or Only Symptomatic Remission

	NO. OF EPISODES	NO. GOING INTO RELAPSE EACH MONTH 1 mo.	2 mos.	3 mos.	4 mos.	5 mos.	6 mos.	RELAPSE TOTAL
Symptomatic and proctoscopic remission	75	11	10	2	5	3	5	35 (47%)
Symptomatic remission only*	71	6	15	10	4	5	5	51 (72%)

*It appears that after complete remission has taken place, relapse is less likely to recur than it is when there are still active inflammatory changes seen on proctoscopy.

normal appearance, marked thickening of the mucosa with a cobblestone appearance or discrete, relatively large ulcers. The coloscopic method is also under current evaluation as a means of detecting early carcinoma in patients with long-standing ulcerative colitis.

INFLUENCE OF VARIOUS FACTORS ON PROGNOSIS

The severity of the clinical picture of ulcerative colitis varies directly with the extent of colonic involvement.[29, 30] Patients with a normal x-ray of the large bowel are seldom subject to incapacitating symptoms or to extracolonic manifestations of ulcerative colitis.[29, 31, 33] There was a striking correlation between a poor prognosis and the extent of involvement of the colon (demonstrated radiologically) in a follow-up study of individuals with ulcerative colitis in the United States Army.[22] Those with universal colitis fared the worst, and those with a normal radiological appearance did the best, while those with partial involvement were intermediate.

A severe attack of ulcerative colitis seems apt to be followed by an unfavorable long-term course. In a study carried out during the presteroid era, Bone et al. found that 70 per cent of patients with severe ulcerative colitis became worse, and 50 per cent required surgical treatment.[7] Our own presteroid experience suggested that the long-term outlook was poor for those patients with fulminating ulcerative colitis who survived under conservative management.[10] Later studies, however, raised a question whether there was an important degree of correlation between the severity of attacks and the subsequent follow-up course.[34, 35] There appears to be general agreement that, when the first referred attack is not severe, the subsequent course of ulcerative colitis cannot be accurately predicted on the basis of the initial severity.

TABLE 1–0 Six-Month Remission Rate on Presteroid Therapy*

EXTENT OF DISEASE	NO. OF EPISODES	NO. ENTERING REMISSION EACH MONTH 1 mo.	2 mos.	3 mos.	4 mos.	5 mos.	6 mos.	TOTAL REMISSION IN 6 MOS.	PER CENT OF 6-MO. REMISSIONS
"Proctitis" (x-ray negative)	40	12	4	8	3	1	0	28	70%
Partial colitis	154	40	26	17	7	8	8	106	69%
Universal colitis	56	17	6	4	4	1	2	34	61%
Totals	250	69	36	29	14	10	10	168	67%

*Remission rates of patients given supportive therapy as related to the anatomical extent of the disease. The remission rate with universal involvement was a little lower than with proctitis or partial colonic involvement.

Various studies have shown that the prognosis for ulcerative colitis is worse early in the course of the disease.[36, 37] Studies of patients treated with steroids demonstrated that patients who were treated during a first attack had a poorer immediate prognosis than those who were treated during relapses.

While a variety of factors appear to have some influence on the severity of attacks of ulcerative colitis, the remission rate over a six-month period is remarkably constant regardless of the extent of anatomical involvement (Table 1–8). During the presteroid era, the incidence of symptomatic remission over a six-month period was between 60 and 70 per cent regardless of whether there was proctitis only, partial colitis or universal colitis.

ATYPICAL AND GRANULOMATOUS COLITIS

An effort has recently been made to separate patients with inflammatory disease of the large bowel into two groups. Lockhart-Mummery and Morson pointed out in 1960 that the pathological findings in patients coming to surgery tended to fit into two categories: a grossly transmural process, microscopically resembling Crohn's disease of the small bowel, or a process primarily involving the superficial layers of the colon.[38] Patients who have been operated upon may thus be classified as having either so-called granulomatous colitis (Crohn's disease of the colon) or nonspecific ulcerative colitis. It is also desirable to differentiate between these two entities in conservatively treated patients.

Attempts to subclassify patients with ulcerative disease of the colon who have not been operated on must be made on the basis of the clinical picture and the radiological, endoscopic and biopsy findings. Many patients who are ultimately demonstrated pathologically to have Crohn's disease present clinical, radiological or endoscopic findings that are unusual in nonspecific ulcerative colitis.[39-43] Nevertheless, much uncertainty still attends our efforts to make a definite distinction clinically between granulomatous colitis and nonspecific ulcerative colitis. There is no simple way in which this can be done with complete precision in the patient who is not operated on, and even in the patient treated surgically there may be disagreement about the pathological findings. At present, a clinical diagnosis of granulomatous colitis is usually based upon a mosaic of clinical, radiological and endoscopic findings. One way to approach this is to isolate a group of individuals with inflammatory bowel disease who have clinical features that are admittedly somewhat unusual for nonspecific ulcerative colitis. Such atypical clinical characteristics may suggest the possibility of a transmural process, but they probably can also occur in some cases of ulcerative colitis. These atypical features include (1) segmental or right-sided colitis with no involvement of the rectum, (2) perianal fistula or abscess, (3) strictures of the large bowel, and (4) a sarcoid-type lesion on rectal biopsy.

A group of 64 patients with some or all of these atypical findings that involve the large bowel but spare the small intestine has been reviewed. These patients were observed in our Ulcerative Colitis Clinic both before and after the introduction of steroids and Azulfidine. We have compared the clinical course of such patients with that observed in patients with ulcerative colitis without any of these atypical features in order to determine whether there is a significant difference in response to medical therapy. The remission and relapse rates have been determined and then compared with the results previously reported for patients with ulcerative colitis. Symptomatic remission has again been defined as the complete absence of symptoms for at least one month.

The incidence of the various atypical aspects in this group was as follows: rectum spared, 29 patients; anal lesion, 17 patients; stricture, 18 patients; sarcoid type of histology, 18 patients.

The remission rates in this group with atypical colitis were not very different from those seen in typical ulcerative colitis. In the atypical group, a remission rate of 50 per cent in six months was observed before the introduction of steroids (Table 1–9). This compared with a six-month symptomatic remission rate of 66 per cent in patients with typical ulcerative colitis limited to the colon.

With steroid therapy, about three quarters of the attacks in the atypical group were terminated within six months—a remission rate that was essentially the same as in typical ulcerative colitis (Table 1–10). The proportion of patients entering remission rapidly was greater than in the presteroid era. In these respects, there was no difference between typical colitis and atypical colitis.

Conservative treatment was interrupted by surgical intervention in 17 of the 64 patients (27 per cent) with atypical findings. This is a somewhat greater proportion than in ulcerative colitis.

TABLE 1–9 Symptomatic Remission Rates During Medical Supportive Therapy (Presteroid) for Typical and Atypical Colitis*

	NO. OF EPISODES	NO. ENTERING REMISSION BY MONTHS		REMISSION TOTAL
		1 to 2 mos.	3 to 6 mos.	
Typical ulcerative colitis	196	73	57	130 (66%)
Atypical ulcerative colitis	76	20	18	38 (50%)

*The six-month remission rate during supportive therapy for atypical colitis was only a little lower than for typical ulcerative colitis.

TABLE 1–10 Symptomatic Remission Rates During Steroid Therapy for Typical and Atypical Colitis*

	NO. OF EPISODES	NO. ENTERING REMISSION BY MONTHS 1 to 2 mos.	3 to 6 mos.	REMISSION TOTAL
Typical ulcerative colitis	54	35	6	41 (76%)
Atypical ulcerative colitis	47	24	10	34 (75%)

*The six-month remission rate during steroid therapy for atypical colitis was the same as for typical ulcerative colitis.

The relapse rate after remission was fairly low (32 per cent) in supportively treated patients with atypical colitis (Table 1–11). This relapse rate is approximately the same as for ulcerative colitis patients not receiving steroid therapy. In the more recently treated patients, in whom steroid therapy was used, the relapse rate was somewhat higher in both groups (Table 1–12).

TABLE 1–11 Relapse Rate After Supportive Treatment*

	NO. OF EPISODES	NO. GOING INTO RELAPSE BY MONTHS 1 to 2 mos.	3 to 6 mos.	RELAPSE TOTAL
Typical ulcerative colitis	70	5	15	20 (28%)
Atypical ulcerative colitis	41	2	11	13 (32%)

*The relapse rate for patients with atypical colitis on supportive therapy was about the same as for those with typical ulcerative colitis.

TABLE 1–12 Relapse Rate After Steroid Remission*

	NO. OF EPISODES	NO. GOING INTO RELAPSE BY MONTHS 1 to 2 mos.	3 to 6 mos.	RELAPSE TOTAL
Typical ulcerative colitis	44	9	12	21 (48%)
Atypical ulcerative colitis	36	3	11	14 (40%)

*The relapse rate for patients with atypical colitis who had entered remission during steroid therapy was essentially the same as for those with typical ulcerative colitis.

At the present time, it appears that an attempt to distinguish between ulcerative colitis and atypical colitis is usually not of major importance with respect to conservative management. It should be noted, however, that toxic dilatation and carcinoma are uncommon in Crohn's disease of the colon. From the standpoint of surgical therapy, the differentiation between the two general types of colitis is much more important; at this time there are reports that suggest that the outlook following surgery may be quite different for these two entities, although this matter is still *subjudice*.[44, 45]

ILEOCOLONIC DISEASE

Patients with inflammatory disease involving both the ileum and the colon often present difficult problems in diagnostic classification and in management. Many of these patients have some of the features listed previously in the discussion of atypical colitis. A large percentage of this group of patients eventually undergo surgery.

For patients not operated on, the classification of individual cases as either nonspecific ulcerative colitis with ileal involvement or granulomatous disease is not always clear-cut; there is considerable overlap in the clinical pictures of the two disorders. Without attempting to make such a classification, one may ask whether involvement of the ileum as well as the colon alters the therapeutic outlook under conservative management.

A group of 57 patients with evidence of both ileal and colonic disease initially was studied to try to solve this question. The clinical course of the group was compared with that of those with typical ulcerative colitis with no ileal involvement. Seventeen of these patients were thought on clinical grounds to have ulcerative colitis with "backwash ileitis," and 40 patients presented some clinical features that were at least consistent with Crohn's disease. Pathological examination of the bowel was eventually carried out in 29 patients, and about half had a pathological picture consistent with granulomatous colitis. The correlation between the clinical impression and the pathological classification was only fair.

On presteroid supportive therapy, the clinical course of most of these patients tended to be of the chronic, unremitting type. Most patients were treated many months without experiencing a sustained period of remission. During the total period of observation, there were 54 episodes for which supportive therapy was used. Remission occurred within six months in only 30 per cent (Table 1–13). This compares unfavorably with typical ulcerative colitis involving the colon but with no ileal disease. The six-month remission rate on supportive treatment for the latter was 66 per cent in this Clinic. Prior to the use of steroids,

TABLE 1–13 Remissions on Supportive Therapy*

	NO. OF EPISODES	NO. ENTERING REMISSION BY MONTHS 1 to 2 mos.	3 to 6 mos.	TOTAL
Ileal and colonic disease	54	10	6	16 (30%)
Ulcerative colitis (colon only)	196	73	57	130 (66%)

*The six-month remission rate for patients with ileal and colonic inflammation treated supportively was considerably lower than that for typical ulcerative colitis without ileal involvement.

surgical intervention was often considered necessary for patients with ileocolonic disease after a prolonged and frustrating trial of medical supportive therapy.

With the introduction of steroid therapy, an abrupt change took place in the response to treatment of patients with ileocolonic inflammatory disease. The six-month remission rate rose to 74 per cent. This rate is almost identical with that for ulcerative colitis limited to the colon (Table 1–14).

The six-month relapse rate after remission induced by steroids was 49 per cent. More than half the relapses took place after steroids had been tapered off or stopped. This is roughly comparable to our experience with typical ulcerative colitis (Table 1–15).

It appears that the results of steroid treatment of ileocolonic disease are very similar to those expected in ulcerative colitis limited to the colon. The remission and relapse rates are similar. Those patients who fail to experience a remission on steroids are now often considered for surgery.

It is also of interest that the pattern of the clinical course is of no assistance in the differential diagnosis. The remission and relapse rates

TABLE 1–14 Remissions on Steroid Therapy*

	NO. OF EPISODES	NO. ENTERING REMISSION BY MONTHS 1 to 2 mos.	3 to 6 mos.	TOTALS
Ileal and colonic disease	53	34	5	39 (74%)
Ulcerative colitis (colon only)	79	46	14	60 (76%)

*The remission rate for patients with ileal and colonic involvement treated with steroids was essentially the same as for patients with typical ulcerative colitis limited to the colon.

TABLE 1–15 **Relapses After Steroid Therapy**

	NO. OF EPISODES	NO. OF RELAPSES BY MONTHS 1 to 2 mos.	3 to 6 mos.	TOTAL IN 6 MOS.	AFTER 6 MOS.
Ileal and colonic disease	43	7 (6*)	14 (10*)	21 (16*)(49%)	22 (10*)
Ulcerative colitis (colon only)	55	14 (12*)	20 (11*)	34 (23*)(62%)	21 (2*)

*Relapses incident to tapering or stopping steroids.

A six-month remission rate of 74 per cent during steroid therapy for ileocolonic inflammation was almost the same as that for ulcerative colitis limited to the colon. Relapse occurred in 49 per cent of patients with ileocolonic inflammation within six months. More than half the relapses took place when steroid therapy had been tapered off or stopped.

were similar for patients who were considered to have ulcerative colitis with "backwash ileitis" and for those with granulomatous disease of the ileum and the colon.

GENERAL CONCLUSIONS

The major points to be derived from these data include the following.

1. More than half of patients undergoing supportive medical treatment for ulcerative colitis will enter remission within six months.
2. The cumulative six-month remission rate is roughly the same with supportive therapy as with steroid therapy.
3. Steroid therapy induces a remission more rapidly in a large number of cases.
4. The relapse rate for patients undergoing supportive medical treatment was lower than for the steroid-treated group.
5. In a group of patients with atypical colitis, the remission and relapse rates were very similar to those for typical ulcerative colitis.
6. The presence of ileal disease results in a lower six-month remission rate with supportive treatment. With steroid therapy, the remission rate is nearly the same as when there is no ileal involvement.

References

1. Hern, J. R. B. Ulcerative colitis. Guy's Hosp. Rep. *81*:322, 1931.
2. Hardy, T. L., and Bulmer, E. Ulcerative colitis, a survey of ninety-five cases. Brit. Med. J. *2*:812, 1933.
3. Hurst, A. F. Prognosis of ulcerative colitis. Lancet *2*:1194, 1935.
4. Kiefer, E. D. Clinical results in the medical treatment of chronic ulcerative colitis. Am. J. Dig. Dis. and Nutrition *3*:56, 1936.

5. Block, M., and Pollard, H. M. Chemotherapy and antibiotics in chronic ulcerative colitis. Gastroenterology *10*:46, 1948.
6. Berkowitz, Z. T. Chloromycetin therapy of chronic ulcerative colitis—a one-year study. Gastroenterology *16*:19, 1950.
7. Bone, F. C., Ruffin, J. M., Baylin, G. J., and Cassel, C. The clinical course of idiopathic ulcerative colitis. South. Med. J. *43*:817, 1950.
8. Rice-Oxley, J. M., and Truelove, S. Ulcerative colitis—course and prognosis. Lancet *1*:663, 1950.
9. Bargen, J. A. Chronic Ulcerative Colitis. Charles C Thomas, Springfield, Ill., 1951.
10. Flood, C. A., Lepore, M. J., Hiatt, R. B., and Karush, A. Prognosis in chronic ulcerative colitis. J. Chronic Dis. *4*:267, 1956.
11. Truelove, S. C., and Witts, L. J. Cortisone in ulcerative colitis—final report on a therapeutic trial. Brit. Med. J. *2*:1041, 1955.
12. Truelove, S. C., and Witts, L. J. Cortisone and corticotropin in ulcerative colitis. Brit. Med. J. *1*:387, 1959.
13. Flood, C. A., and Sweeting, J. Results of Medical Therapy in Ulcerative Colitis. *In* Modern Gastroenterology. Gregor, O., and Riedl. O., eds. Schattauer Verlag. Stuttgart, 1969, pp. 1004–1006.
14. Svartz, N. Salazopyrin, a new sulfanilamide preparation. A. Therapeutic results in rheumatoid polyarthritis. B. Therapeutic results in ulcerative colitis. C. Toxic manifestations in treatment with sulfanilamide preparations. Acta Med. Scand. *110*:577, 1942.
15. Holst, J. E. Chemotherapeutical treatment of severe colitis and proctitis. Acta Med. Scand. *113*:109, 1943.
16. Svartz, N. The treatment of 124 cases of ulcerative colitis with salazopyrine and attempts of desensitization in cases of hypersensitiveness to sulfa. Acta Med. Scand. (Suppl.) *206*:465, 1948.
17. Leonard-Jones, J. E., Longmore, A. J., Newell, A. C., Wilson, C. W. E., and Jones, F. A. An assessment of prednisone, salazopyrine and topical hydrocortisone hemisuccinate used as out-patient treatment for ulcerative colitis. Gut:*1*:212, 1961.
18. Dick, A. P., Grayson, M. J., Carpenter, R. G., and Petrie, A. Controlled trial of sulphasalazine in the treatment of ulcerative colitis. Gut 5:437, 1964.
19. Misiewicz, J. J., Leonard-Jones, J. E., Connell, A. M., Baron, J. H., and Jones, F. Controlled trial of sulphasalazine in maintenance therapy for ulcerative colitis. Lancet *1*:185, 1965.
20. Bargen, J. A. Chronic Ulcerative Colitis—A Life Long Study. Charles C Thomas, Springfield, Ill., 1969, p. 45.
21. Watts, J. M., de Dombal, F. T., Watkinson, G., and Goligher, J. C. Long term prognosis of ulcerative colitis. Brit. Med. J. *1*:1447, 1966.
22. Nefziger, M. D., and Acheson, E. D. Ulcerative colitis in the United States Army in 1944. Follow-up with particular reference to mortality in cases and controls. Gut *4*:183, 1963.
23. Edwards, F. C., and Truelove, S. C. The course and prognosis of ulcerative colitis. III. Complications. Gut 5:1, 1964.
24. Goligher, J. C., de Dombal, F. T., Watts, J. M., and Watkinson, G. Ulcerative Colitis. The Williams & Wilkins Co., Baltimore, Md., 1968.
25. Bonnevie, O., Binder, V., Anthonisen, P., and Riis, P. The prognosis of ulcerative colitis. Scand. J. Gastroenterol. 9:81, 1974.
26. Riis, P. Therapeutic influences in the prognosis of ulcerative colitis. Scand. J. Gastroenterol. 9:1, 1974.
27. Crohn, B. B., and Rosenberg, H. Sigmoidoscopic picture of chronic ulcerative colitis (nonspecific). Amer. J. Med. Sci. *170*:220, 1925.
28. Wright, R., and Truelove, S. C. Serial rectal biopsy in ulcerative colitis during the course of a controlled therapeutic trial of various diets. Amer. J. Dig. Dis. *11*:847, 1966.
29. Bockus, H. L., Roth, J. L. A., Buchman, E., Kalser, M., Staub, W. R., Finkelstein, A., and Valdes-Dapena, A. Life history of non-specific ulcerative colitis. Relation of prognosis to anatomic and clinical varieties. Gastroenterology *86*:549, 1956.
30. Watts, J. M., de Dombal, F. T., Watkinson, G., and Goligher, J. C. Early course of ulcerative colitis. Gut *7*:16, 1966.

31. Leonard-Jones, G. W., Cooper, A. C., Newell, A. C., Wilson, C. W. E., and Jones, F. A. Observations on idiopathic proctitis. Gut 3:201, 1962.
32. Sparberg, M., Fennessy, J., and Kirsner, J. B. Ulcerative proctitis and mild ulcerative colitis. A study of 220 patients. Medicine 45:391, 1966.
33. Nugent, F. W., Veidenheimer, M. C., Zuberi, S., Garabedian, M., and Parikh, N. K. Clinical course of ulcerative proctosigmoiditis. Amer. J. Dig. Dis. *15*:321, 1970.
34. Jalan, K. N., Prescott, R. J., Sircus, W. Z., Card, W. I., McManus, J. P. A., Falconer, C. W. A., Small, W. P., Smith, A. N., and Bruce, J. An experience of ulcerative colitis. II. Short term outcome. Gastroenterology *59*:589, 1970.
35. Jalan, K. N., Prescott, R. J., Sircus, W. Z., Card, W. I., McManus, J. P. A., Falconer, C. W. A., Small, W. P., Smith, A. N., and Bruce, J. An experience of ulcerative colitis. III. Long term outcome. Gastroenterology *59*:598, 1970.
36. Carleson, R., Fristedt, B., and Philipson, J. Ulcerative colitis. A follow-up investigation of a 20 year primary material. Acta Med. Scand. *172*:647, 1962.
37. Edwards, F. C., and Truelove, S. C. The course and prognosis of ulcerative colitis. Gut 4:299, 1963.
38. Lockhart-Mummery, H. E., and Morson, B. C. Crohn's disease (regional enteritis) of the large intestine and its distinction from ulcerative colitis. Gut *1*:87, 1960.
39. Linder, A. E., Marshak, R. H., and Wolf, B. S. Granulomatous colitis. Clinical study. New Eng. J. Med. *269*:379, 1963.
40. Janowitz, H. D., Linder, A. E., and Marshak, R. Granulomatous colitis; Crohn's disease of the colon. J. A. M. A. *191*:825, 1965.
41. McGovern,, V. J., and Goulston, S. J. Crohn's disease of the colon. Gut 9:164, 1968.
42. Schachter, H., Goldstein, M. J., Rappaport, H., Fennessy, M. B., and Kirsner, J. B. Ulcerative and "granulomatous" colitis. Validity of differential diagnostic criteria. A study of 100 patients treated by total colectomy. Ann. Intern. Med. *72*:841, 1970.
43. Nelson, J. A., Margulis, A. R., Goldberg, H. I., and Lawson, T. L. Granulomatous colitis; significance of involvement of the terminal ileum. Gastroenterology *64*:1071, 1973.
44. Korelitz, B. I. Clinical course, late results, and pathological nature of inflammatory disease of the colon initially sparing the rectum. Gut *8*:281, 1967.
45. Glotzer, D. J., Gardner, R. C., Goldman, H., Hinrichs, H. R., Rosen, H., and Zetzel, L. Comparative features and course of ulcerative and granulomatous colitis. New Eng. J. Med. *282*:582, 1970.

Chapter Two

VARIABLE EFFECTS OF PSYCHOTHERAPY IN ULCERATIVE COLITIS

The importance of providing emotional support to the patient with ulcerative colitis is generally recognized by both gastroenterologists and psychiatrists. It is claimed by some that such assurance is best provided by a sympathetic internist, and that the assistance of the psychiatrist is usually unnecessary in the management of patients with ulcerative colitis. On the other hand, as if to challenge an oversimplification, many patients with ulcerative colitis spontaneously seek psychiatric help despite the neutrality or the skepticism of their internists.

The difficulty in justifying the value of psychotherapy is demonstrated in the presentation that follows. During the earlier years of the Columbia ulcerative colitis project, patients were assigned to psychiatrists more or less indiscriminately, with little concern for specific criteria about their treatability. No distinction could be made about the type of psychotherapeutic intervention that might best serve a particular patient. Furthermore, no thought was given to pairing the personality of the therapist to the personality of the patient, a subject that has only recently been seriously taken into consideration.

As a result, it has not been possible to establish the value of psychotherapy to the total program of treatment for ulcerative colitis with any consistency. The presentations in this chapter and in Chapters Four and Five describe our efforts to focus on the factors that must be taken into account if psychotherapy is to be useful.

We begin with parallel studies of two large series of cases. In study *A*, 50 patients were selected by two criteria. First, their records of periodic follow-up examinations after psychotherapy had been started were the most complete ones available. Second, the patients had received some kind of psychotherapy from psychiatrists or psychiatric residents. Fully matched controls were not used. The control population to which the psychotherapeutically treated patients were compared for somatic and symptomatic changes consisted of patients with illness of equivalent severity who had undergone no psychotherapy. Attempts could not be made to match test cases and controls according to psychopathology, since study *A* was essentially a retrospective one and few of the controls had been evaluated psychiatrically.

The first effort to define the effects of psychiatric differences on the outcome of a treatment that included psychotherapy was mainly concerned with the significance of schizophrenia to the prognosis. This second series of 57, *B*, included several of the patients studied in the first series, and it also had a control population matched case for case for age, sex and severity of colon disease. About one third of this control group, however, had undergone a psychiatric evaluation. The remainder had not been diagnosed psychiatrically apparently because they did not display overt psychiatric symptoms. Indeed, the control group appeared to include fewer schizophrenics than did the test group and, psychiatrically at least, was not as ill.

The third and most sharply focused study, described in detail later, dealt with the psychological factors involved in the predisposition to ulcerative colitis and with the responsiveness of different patients to different kinds of therapeutic intervention.

Studies *A* and *B* led to somewhat different conclusions about the value of psychotherapy. These contradictory findings are typical of the variable claims made for psychotherapy in the literature, in which one report praises psychotherapy and another damns it, or at best considers it hardly worth the trouble. One important reason for such conflicting views has been the absence of well-defined criteria for selecting the patients suitable for psychotherapy, for choosing the most compatible psychotherapist and, finally, for adapting the nature of the therapy to the psychological capacities and limitations of each patient. When the approach to the ulcerative colitis sufferer is individualized in this way, the outcome of discriminately applied psychotherapy becomes more reliably positive. There will, of course, be patients who may need no psychotherapy, and there will be those in whom it cannot affect the somatic illness. In this latter group, it may nevertheless still help to reduce the personal and social disability caused by the colitis. Until a specific etiology can be discovered and a specific therapy devised, an objective and unbiased attitude toward psychotherapy will do much to provide a more optimistic future for the colitis victim.

SERIES A*

The clinical course of 50 patients with inflammatory disease of the colon was monitored by periodic follow-up visits after they had been

*The analysis of the data from this study is presented here for the first time.

TABLE 2–1 Results of Psychotherapy in Ulcerative Colitis (Series A)

FIRST REFERRED ATTACK					REMITTERS AFTER FIRST ATTACK		
Outcome of Attack	**No. of Patients**	**Average Severity**	**Average Duration (months)**	**Deaths**	**Outcome for Remitters**	**No. of Patients**	**Average Duration (months)**
Operations	7	3.0	58.7[a]	0	Still in remission	0	
Lost before remission	7	2.7	18.8[a]		Lost in remission	8	43.6[a]
Data incomplete	1				Data incomplete	3	
Went into remission	38	2.7	9.2[b]	—	Followed to next attack	25	17.0[d]
Total	43			0	Total	36[c]	

SECOND ATTACK					REMITTERS AFTER SECOND ATTACK		
Outcome of Attack	**No. of Patients**	**Average Severity**	**Average Duration (months)**	**Deaths**	**Outcome for Remitters**	**No. of Patients**	**Average Duration (months)**
Operations	2	3.0	2.5[a]	0	Still in remission	1	
Lost before remission	2	2.0	6.0[a]		Lost in remission	7	53.0[a]
Data incomplete	2				Data incomplete	1	
Went into remission	22	1.8	3.9[e]	0	Followed to next attack	15	14.8[f]
Total	28			0	Total	24	

	THIRD ATTACK				REMITTERS AFTER THIRD ATTACK		
Outcome of Attack	No. of Patients	Average Severity	Average Duration (months)	Deaths	Outcome for Remitters	No. of Patients	Average Duration (months)
Operations	1	3.0	1.0[a]	0	Still in remission	0	
Lost before remission	3	2.5	9.5[a]		Lost in remission	3	29.0[a]
Data incomplete	2				Data incomplete	2	
Went into remission	10	1.7	3.5[g]		Followed to next attack	7	9.3[h]
Total	16			0	Total	12	

[a]Duration to loss or surgery.
[b]Range – 1 to 90 months.
[c]Includes 28 patients followed to remission after the first referred attack, 1 patient with incomplete data for the first attack, and 7 patients who entered the study while in remission.
[d]Range – 2 to 58 months.
[e]Range – 1 to 12 months.
[f]Range – 1 to 42 months.
[g]Range – 1 to 12 months.
[h]Range – 1 to 14 months.

placed in psychotherapy. The patients remained under continuous medical supervision. The results of this study were recorded by the same methods described in Chapter One. They have been presented in part in previous communications.[1–3] The present series of 50 patients was selected from a larger group who had received psychotherapy because their follow-up medical records were almost complete and were continuous.

The group consisted of 15 males and 35 females. Four patients were black; 21 were Jewish. The average age was 27.8 years at the time of the initial visit, and the average duration of the disease was 4.5 years.

There were 15 patients in the group who had total colonic involvement as seen on radiological and proctoscopic examination. Twenty-one had partial involvement initially; four later progressed to total involvement. Three patients in the series had proctitis only, the radiological examination having been normal.

In retrospect, 11 of the 50 patients might be considered to have had features that were atypical for nonspecific ulcerative colitis; they could therefore be interpreted to have had granulomatous colitis. Seven of these 11 patients had segmental involvement of the colon, three had strictures of the colon or rectum, and one had a granulomatous type of inflammatory process demonstrated by biopsy.

Seventeen of the 50 patients received steroids, corticotropin or Azulfidine at some point in their clinical course. The impact of these medications on the clinical course of the patients is discussed later.

Each of the 50 patients was placed in a program of psychotherapy that consisted of a minimum of eight psychotherapeutic sessions.

The outcome for all patients is summarized in Table 2–1. A gradual attrition took place in this group, as a number of individuals required surgery or were lost to follow-up. The original group of 50 patients had dwindled to 28 by the second referred attack and to 16 by the third attack. A total of 10 patients required surgery; seven were operated upon during the first referred attack. Eleven patients were lost to follow-up while in an attack and presumably sought medical care elsewhere. A large number of patients, 18, were lost to follow-up while in remission. Most of these patients had been in remission a long time before they were lost to the series. Presumably, lack of symptoms was the reason for the failure to reappear for examination in some instances.

It should also be noted that 7 of the 50 patients are not listed under the first referred attack because they entered psychiatric treatment during a period of symptomatic remission. These seven patients are first included in the tabulation under the first remission.

The first referred attack in this series of patients was often long, averaging 9.2 months for those patients who entered remission. The second and third attacks were of substantially shorter duration, with averages of 3.9 and 3.5 months, respectively, for those patients who remained under observation until remission had taken place.

The first referred attack was also more severe than subsequent attacks. Most patients were incapacitated by their symptoms during that period. Second and third attacks were substantially milder, and most patients had only mild or moderate symptoms.

Remissions between each attack averaged roughly more than one year in duration. Following the first referred attack, the average duration of remission was 17 months; the second remission averaged 14.8 months; and the third averaged 9.3 months. The latter figure may be somewhat misleading because of the small number of patients involved.

Comparison of Clinical Course of Patients with and without Psychotherapy

The results from the 50 patients treated by psychotherapy were compared with those from 81 patients given medical supportive therapy alone. The 81 patients selected for comparison are those described in Chapter One. Patients who had proctitis alone were deleted from the original group of 103 patients, reducing the number to 81. This was done to make the group more closely comparable to the psychiatrically treated group, which contained only three patients with proctitis.

The distributions of patients in the psychiatrically treated series and of those who received medical supportive therapy were approximately the same with respect to sex, age and race (Table 2–2). The proportions of patients with partial or total colonic involvement and with atypical features were also similar for the two groups. The psychiatrically treated group included three patients with proctitis, while the

TABLE 2–2 Comparison of Symptomatically Treated Series and Psychiatrically Treated Series

	SYMPTOMATIC TREATMENT	PSYCHIATRIC TREATMENT
No. of patients	81	50
Sex	M 33	M 15
	F 48	F 35
Average age	37.9 yrs.	27.8 yrs.
Age range	15–86 yrs.	12–52 yrs.
Average duration	4.5 yrs.	4.5 yrs.
Duration range	(1–20 yrs.)	(1–20 yrs.)
Extent of disease (Typical ulcerative colitis)		
Proctitis	0	3
Partial	48	21
Total	16	15
Atypical colitis	17	11
Treated with steroids or Azulfidine	0	17

other group had none. The psychiatrically treated group contained a few more patients younger than 20 years of age but had none older than 70.

A comparison of the psychiatrically treated patients with those who did not receive psychotherapy indicates that the former had a more severe first referred attack (Table 2–3). The average duration of the first referred attack was about twice as long for the psychiatrically treated patients. The severity rating for the first attack was 2.7 for the psychiatrically treated group as compared with 2.3 for the other group, indicating that a larger proportion of patients who received psychotherapy were incapacitated during the first referred attack.

Surgical intervention was carried out in a somewhat larger proportion of patients in the psychiatrically treated group during the first referred attack. It is of interest, however, that operation was usually delayed for a long period before it was eventually carried out in the psychiatric group. This reflects the fact that a period of trial psychotherapy often preceded the final decision for surgical intervention in this sicker group. The proportion of patients who were lost to follow-up while still in the first referred attack was about the same for both groups, although the length of follow-up to the time of the loss was greater in the psychiatrically treated group.

The first referred attack eventually ended in symptomatic remission in about two thirds of each group (28 of 43 patients vs. 57 of 81 controls). The duration of the first remission for each group was about the same (17 months for patients vs. 15.8 months for controls).

The average duration of the second referred attack was approximately the same for both groups but was slightly shorter in the psychiat-

TABLE 2–3 Supportive vs. Psychiatric Therapy in Ulcerative Colitis*

	FIRST ATTACK		**SECOND ATTACK**		**THIRD ATTACK**	
	Support.	**Psych.**	**Support.**	**Psych.**	**Support.**	**Psych.**
Average duration of attack (months)	4.8	9.2	5.4	3.9	4.8	3.5
Average severity of attack (scale of 0–3)	2.3	2.7	1.5	1.8	1.7	1.7
	FIRST REMISSION		**SECOND REMISSION**		**THIRD REMISSION**	
	Support.	**Psych.**	**Support.**	**Psych.**	**Support.**	**Psych.**
Average duration of remission	15.8	17.0	12.6	14.8	20.0	9.3

*Comparison of average duration and maximal severity of attacks and duration of remissions in 81 patients treated by supportive therapy alone and in 50 patients who received psychotherapy. The first referred attack was worse in both duration and severity in the group receiving psychotherapy. The above figures are derived from the data in Tables 1–1 and 2–1.

rically treated patients. The third attack was also somewhat shorter in the psychiatrically treated patients. There was little difference in the average duration of the second remission (14.8 months for patients vs. 12.5 months for controls). The third remission was longer in the treated group, but the number of patients involved is quite small.

Fifteen of the 50 psychiatrically treated patients received steroids or corticotropin at some time during the period of observation. The question arises, how much impact did these hormones have on the clinical course? Some effect is apparent, although the relative number of patients who manifested improvement is small. Eleven patients received steroids or corticotropin at some time during the first referred attack. The treatment with steroids seemed to induce remission in four of these patients. Similarly, seven patients received hormonal therapy during the second attack, with remission occurring in three. Only two patients received steroids for the third attack, and both entered remission.

Four patients also received Azulfidine during four episodes in the course of their observation. This drug appeared to induce a remission in two of the four patients. It was not used prophylactically in this study.

In summary, steroids, corticotropin or Azulfidine appears to have induced a remission in four patients in this series during the first referred attack, in three patients during the second referred attack and in three patients during the third attack. This is a total of 12 remissions incident to drug therapy during the first three observed attacks and constitutes 20 per cent of the remissions observed in the psychiatrically treated patients during the first three attacks.

Follow-up by Years

An analysis of the follow-up of psychiatrically treated patients in terms of patient years reveals a gradual improvement year by year (Fig. 2–1). The average severity of symptoms in the first years was in the semi-incapacitated range (2.4). Over the succeeding years the average patient had only mild to moderate symptoms. Progressive improvement for the series is seen over several years. It should be reemphasized that the initial referred attack is apt to be more severe than average regardless of the treatment used; this may in part account for these observations.

A comparison of the psychiatrically treated group to the group who received simple medical supportive treatment reveals that both series experienced progressive improvement over the years. The psychiatrically treated group fared better in terms of average severity of symptoms as the years progressed. As seen in Figure 2–1, the per annum severity of symptoms was substantially less in the fourth to seventh year of follow-up.

In summary, psychotherapy combined with supportive medical therapy in this series of patients seems to have enabled a group of indi-

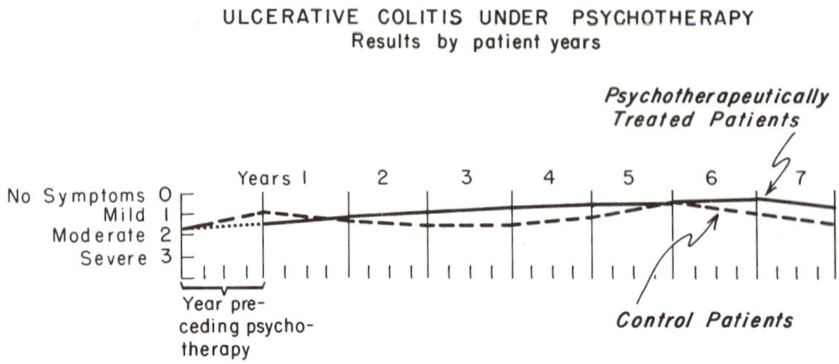

Figure 2–1 Comparison of average severity of symptoms year by year between a group of patients [Series A] treated supportively without psychotherapy and a group treated both medically and psychotherapeutically, as described in the text. Each point on the curve was derived by calculating the average severity for those patients who remained under conservative management each year. The degree of severity of symptoms for each patient year was calculated by finding an average for the year.

viduals with severe symptoms to carry on under conservative management and to enter symptomatic remission. Subsequent attacks in these patients were no more severe and, in fact, tended to be of slightly shorter duration than in a series of patients who did not receive psychotherapy. It appears that psychotherapy helped diminish the severity of symptoms during subsequent flare-ups of the disease. The duration of symptomatic remission was virtually the same both in psychiatrically treated patients and in those who received only medical supportive therapy.

This study suggests that the addition of psychotherapy to the management of the more seriously ill patient with ulcerative colitis helps the patient to adjust to the illness and may be instrumental in enabling him or her to carry on under conservative treatment to a point of remission. It may also contribute somewhat to reducing the severity of subsequent attacks. Our statistical data from this group of patients, however, do not show convincing evidence that psychotherapy increases the duration of remission in ulcerative colitis.

SERIES B

Fifty-seven patients who received no less than three months of psychotherapy were matched case for case for age, sex, severity of the disease process and the comparable use of steroids, to controls who received no psychotherapy.[3] The follow-up period for all patients was five or more years. No patient had been ill for fewer than five years; the average duration of the disease in both study and control groups was 15 years. Both groups consisted of 32 females and 25 males.

The physiological criteria for rating the severity of the disease process in the colon were described in Chapter One. Because of the significance of the organic severity of the disease, treated and untreated groups were further matched according to their symptomatic and proctoscopic ratings in the first recorded year of disease and according to the extent of the pathological involvement of the colon, whether total, segmental or partial, at that same time.

The psychological criteria for the psychiatric diagnoses are set forth in the Diagnostic and Statistical Manual of Mental Disorders, published by the American Psychiatric Association in 1952. Psychometric tests, including the Wechsler-Bellevue, Rorschach and Thematic Apperception Tests, were administered to clarify doubtful diagnoses.

A modification of a scale introduced by H. R. Klein was used to evaluate psychological changes in certain aspects of life function before and after psychotherapy.[4] The areas rated were career (work or school), sex, marriage, family and self-esteem. Ratings were made on a 1 to 5 scale, 5 indicating normal function and 1, poorest function. The criteria for rating "career" performance illustrate the construction of the scales used to compare overt behavioral changes:

Rating 1: Incapable of any work.
Rating 2: Unable to work more than half-time, with minimal pleasure or gratification.
Rating 3: Works most of the time fairly effectively, possibly below the appropriate level of training, but with limited pleasure and gratification.
Rating 4: Works steadily and effectively, with minor periods of dysfunction and few periods of clearly reduced pleasure.
Rating 5: Able to enjoy sustained satisfactory and harmonious work (or school) adjustment, with a high degree of pleasure and gratification.

The psychological response to psychotherapy was measured by comparing the pretreatment rating with the post-treatment rating. For ex-

TABLE 2–4 Psychological Response to Psychotherapy

AREAS OF FUNCTION	PREPSYCHO-THERAPY RATING	POSTPSYCHO-THERAPY RATING	SCORE
Career	2	5	+3
Sexual and marital	2	4	+2
Family	2	3	+1
Self-esteem	2	5	+3
Total change			+9

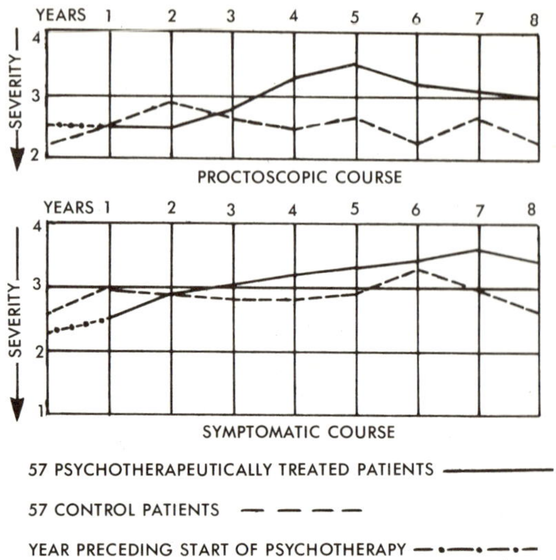

Figure 2–2 Proctoscopic and symptomatic ratings of psychotherapeutically treated patients and control patients. Surgical cases and deaths are not rated as failures.

ample, in the patient described in Table 2–4, the total change would be +9, an excellent psychological response. This patient had moved from fair functioning in all life areas to good functioning in all but the "family" area.

The series as a whole was divided into categories of responses, ranging from "excellent" to "poor," according to the numerical ratings (Table 2–5).

Figures 2–2 to 2–5 illustrate how the proctoscopic and symptomatic course of the illness was projected over an eight-year period. The patients averaged three proctoscopic examinations per year. The first year on the chart precedes the start of psychotherapy; the remaining seven years are those following its inception.

A certain pattern of responsiveness to treatment was observed in this series of patients. During the first year of psychotherapy, the treated patients did poorer as a group and rated consistently lower than the control group, but by the third year, a sustained improvement became apparent. By the time of final observation, the treated group showed considerably greater improvement both symptomatically and protoscopically than the control group, which showed no improvement from its

TABLE 2–5 Scoring of Psychological Response

SCORE	RESPONSE
Plus 7 and above	Excellent
Plus 4 to 6	Good
Plus 2 to 3	Fair to moderate
0 to plus 1	No change
Minus 1 and below	Poor

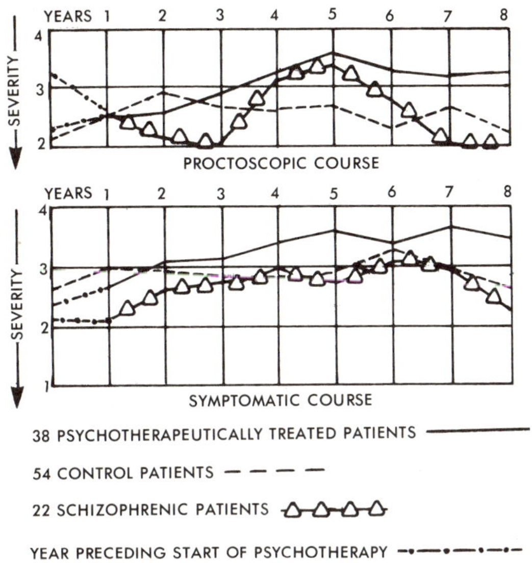

Figure 2–3 Proctoscopic and symptomatic ratings of psychotherapeutically treated patients and control patients, with schizophrenic patients removed and charted as a separate group. Surgical cases and deaths are not rated as failures.

initial symptomatic rating and made but a minimal gain proctoscopically.

The psychiatric diagnostic factors recognized in series *B* patients consisted of psychoneurosis, personality disorder and schizophrenia. Nineteen patients were considered schizophrenic, 3 were psychoneurotic and 34 suffered from personality disorders. One, an adolescent, was undiagnosed. The selection factor in this series weighted patients toward severe psychopathology that was obvious to the relatively untrained eyes of nonpsychiatrists. The more noticeably disturbed the patient was, the

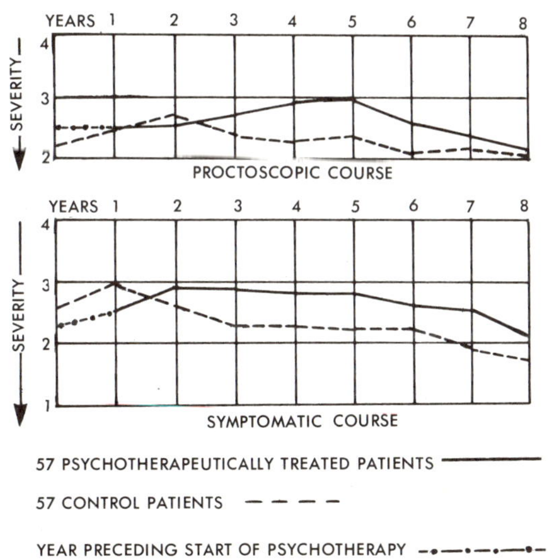

Figure 2–4 Proctoscopic and symptomatic ratings of all psychotherapeutically treated patients and control patients, including surgical cases and deaths, which are considered to be failures.

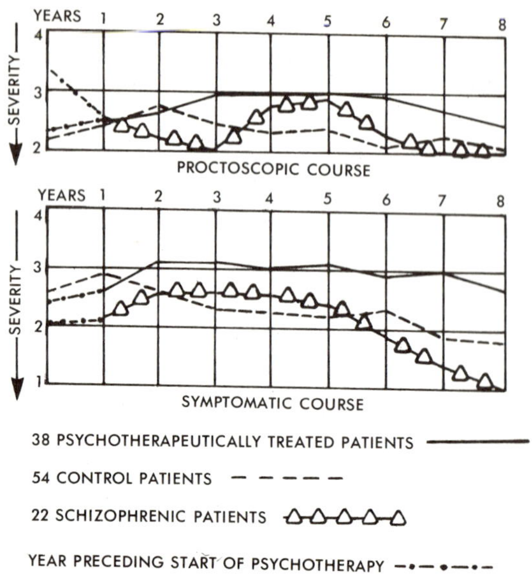

Figure 2–5 Proctoscopic and symptomatic ratings of psychotherapeutically treated patients and control patients, with schizophrenic patients removed and charted as a separate group. Surgical cases and deaths are included as failures.

more certain he was to be referred to the psychiatrist, and the greater the population of emotionally very ill patients in series *B*. These proportions cannot, therefore, be claimed to represent the natural distribution of psychological illnesses among all ulcerative colitis patients. There were, for example, only 3 known cases of schizophrenia among the controls. Nevertheless, this "biased" sample did demonstrate an important correlation between gross psychiatric diagnosis and somatic prognosis in patients treated medically and psychiatrically.

Fluctuations in the proctoscopic and symptomatic courses were more pronounced among the schizophrenic patients. It was not possible to conclude from the relatively small number of patients with schizophrenia that the mental disorder produced a greater tendency toward exacerbation, although this seems likely to be true.

Proctoscopically, the treated group as a whole scored significantly higher by the last recorded year, while the controls remained essentially unchanged (Fig. 2–4). The schizophrenic cases, when separated from the rest of the treated group, were decidedly worse (Fig. 2–5).

Symptomatically, the treated group as a whole fared better than the control group. The nonschizophrenic treated group did much better than either the control group or the schizophrenic patients, improving 1.1 points to a 3.5 rating, which denoted almost complete absence of symptoms. The control group remained relatively unchanged.

There was other evidence of the serious impact of psychosis on the somatic prognosis. In the psychiatrically treated group of patients, 32 per cent of the schizophrenics died, and 37 per cent underwent major surgery. These figures compared with a death rate of 8 per cent and a surgical rate of 21 per cent for the nonschizophrenic portion of the treated group.

The use of steroids reduced the mortality rate by 50 per cent in both treated and control patients.

As for the general comparisons between the psychotherapeutically treated group and the control group in terms of extent of colonic involvement, there seemed to be greater improvement in the treated group with respect to the subsequent severity of somatic disease. Twenty-six per cent of the treated patients ultimately developed total involvement of the colon, as compared with 40 per cent of the controls. Surgical and death rates for patients with total colitis were equal in treated and control cases. Among those with partial and segmental colonic involvement, the combined surgical and mortality rate was 37 per cent for the psychiatrically treated group, as compared with 57 per cent for the control group. These figures suggest that psychotherapy helps to prevent progression of the disease to the point at which changes in the colon become irreversible.

Comparison of the findings and implications in series *A* to those in series *B* underlines their considerable differences. In *A* no clearly significant effects of psychotherapy were found. In *B*, on the other hand, not only did treated patients do better than their matched controls, but also differences in psychopathology were found to have a significant impact upon the prognosis.

Two sets of factors may account for these contradictory conclusions. In series *A*, no data were cited to indicate the extent and the nature of the *psychiatric problem*. There was no reliable way to determine the proportion of emotional problems that were more or less likely to be helped by psychotherapy. No discernible or precise criteria were available for comparative purposes. Series *B* had some advantage in this regard—not only had all the psychotherapeutically treated patients been evaluated diagnostically, but two thirds of the controls had also been examined, however superficially, by a psychiatrist. Thirty-seven controls received no psychiatric diagnosis simply because they displayed no overt symptoms. Three, however, were diagnosed as schizophrenic, 3 as psychoneurotic and 14 as having personality disorders. The control group in series *B* was apparently less emotionally disturbed than the treated patients.

A second group of factors may have even more significance in accounting for the contradictory findings. Series *A* included a large number of treated patients whose psychotherapy records were skimpy or nonexistent. Many more of the series *B* psychotherapists were supervised psychiatrists who were postgraduate students in the Columbia Psychoanalytic Clinic for Training and Research. They were required to keep detailed process records of each session for discussion with their supervisors. Thus, the series *B* patients tended to have a more sophisticated group of psychotherapists whose diagnoses and treatment techniques were closely checked. One cannot escape the suspicion that treated series *B* patients may have enjoyed a considerable advantage over many of those in series *A*, whose therapists were in general less adequately trained and less rigorously supervised.

It is these two factors that, to our knowledge, have not been examined in reports purporting to disprove claims for the value of psychotherapy. They have not reported the nature of or the criteria used for the psychiatric evaluations of treated patients, and they have not reported the level of skill in psychotherapy of the therapists whose cases they compare with their untreated controls.

Neither series *A* nor series *B* examined psychological factors other than in diagnosis. The issues involved in the psychotherapeutic interventions actually used and in the relative value of various techniques of therapy for different types of psychological disturbances were not considered in either study, nor for that matter in any other published report about the treatment of ulcerative colitis.

We discuss both issues in Chapters Four and Five to help reduce the number of or obviate futile debates about the usefulness of psychotherapy in the management of many cases of ulcerative colitis.

References

1. Daniels, G. E., O'Connor, J. F., Karush, A., Moses, L., Flood, C. A., and Lepore, M. Three decades in the observation and treatment of ulcerative colitis. Psychosom. Med. *24*:85, 1962.
2. O'Connor, J. F., Daniels, G., Flood, C., Karush, A., Moses, L., and Stern, L. O. An evaluation of the effectiveness of psychotherapy in the treatment of ulcerative colitis. Ann. Intern. Med., *60*:587, 1964.
3. Karush, A., Daniels, G. E., O'Connor, J. F., and Stern, L. O. The response to psychotherapy in chronic ulcerative colitis. Psychosom. Med. *31*:201, 1969.
4. Klein, H. R. A study of changes occurring in patients during and after psychoanalytic treatment. *In* Current Approaches to Psychoanalysis. Hoch, P., and Zubin, J., eds. Grune & Stratton, Inc., New York, 1960, 151.

Chapter Three

A REVIEW OF THE PSYCHOSOMATIC LITERATURE ON CHRONIC ULCERATIVE COLITIS

EARLY CONTRIBUTIONS

The presence of psychological factors significant to ulcerative colitis was first discovered during a psychological investigation of disease carried out by the Constitution Clinic of the Department of Medicine at the Presbyterian Hospital (New York), under the general direction of Dr. George Draper. Attention was drawn to several patients with ulcerative colitis who were admitted to the hospital wards.

The initial study was conducted by Cecil D. Murray, who in 1930 published two reports on the first cases of ulcerative colitis to be studied from a psychological viewpoint.[36, 37] Murray described "a well marked time relationship between the outbreak of an emotional disturbance and the onset of symptoms." These conclusions soon stimulated further investigations at Columbia-Presbyterian Medical Center and elsewhere.

Precipitating psychological stress seemed to play a surprisingly important role in the four cases. Symptoms of bloody diarrhea appeared on the day of one young woman's secret marriage. Blood appeared in the stool of a 27-year-old woman after interest was shown by her first suitor and the possibility of marriage threatened to become a reality. More serious symptoms of ulcerative colitis occurred when her engagement to another man led her closer and closer to marriage. A 33-year-old man developed diarrhea a month or two after starting a relationship with a girl in his neighborhood. Two years later, an attack of severe colitis that required hospitalization was precipitated by his public engagement to be married.

Murray published a second paper in 1930 with a more detailed psychological analysis of a case. The patient's symptoms appeared after she and her lover registered as man and wife at a European hotel. Murray was able to demonstrate the relationship between suppressed rage and her symptoms. He stressed that an early infantile fixation involving her dead mother had sensitized the patient to fears of dying for any transgression. Murray's patients were marked by emotional immaturity, and he emphasized the infantile connection between fear and diarrhea. The most frequent conflict in his cases involved an excessive attachment to the mother that was threatened by the desire to marry. All seven men in his series were single and were abnormally attached to their mothers or, in one case, to an older sister. Murray stressed that it is not usually a sudden fright that causes the difficulty, but rather a new, continuing situation that keeps the patient in a constant state of apprehension. He felt that the psychological factors in ulcerative colitis are similar to those long recognized in simple diarrhea and mucous colitis. Murray's early experience led to the use of psychotherapy for ulcerative colitis patients on the hospital wards.

Albert J. Sullivan, an internist in New Haven, undertook the psychotherapeutic treatment of ulcerative colitis, consulting a psychiatrist only in severe cases. He reported his findings in 30 patients followed over seven years.[3, 47, 48]

Five of seven young men had abnormal emotional attachments to their mothers, similar to those Murray had observed. The onset of diarrhea was related to pregnancy or childbirth in two women and in one man; in two other cases there appeared to be a chronological relationship, although he could identify no clear psychological connection between specific events and illness. Sullivan found that the onset of symptoms was often precipitated by an emotional disturbance, and he noted that it might take weeks before one gained the patient's confidence enough for specific problems of etiological importance to become apparent.

The difficulty in eliciting the crucial factors, Sullivan stated, "would lead one into endless investigation of the psychoanalyst if it were not for the fact that there is an amazingly clear chronological association between emotional episodes and the onset of bloody diarrhea." Sullivan also pointed out the great aid this can be to therapy. He reported that in 11 of 15 cases, the emotionally charged event was followed by bloody diarrhea within 24 to 48 hours.

Sullivan observed that as the nuclear conflict was approached, a patient's symptoms often became temporarily exacerbated, with fever, increased diarrhea and vomiting.

This development of symptoms also included emotional changes. Sullivan's patients seemed to suppress the usual expressions of anger, despair and triumph, and were often considered nonchalant and unemotional by their families. With psychotherapy, however, a loosening of emotional expression would take place that was not always approved by their parents and spouses.

In the bulk of Sullivan's cases, the disease began between the ages of 20 and 30, when the person was called on to assume adult responsibilities. In the 30 cases reviewed by Sullivan's group, there was no evidence of even one successful marriage. Sullivan expressed the opinion that, from his experience, psychogenic factors frequently are the main cause of the disease, and he observed that psychotherapy may produce striking results when other therapies fail.

Sullivan reported that not infrequently there was a history of constipation, an important early symptom in some patients. He contrasted the ulcerative colitis patients with the peptic ulcer patients, whom he described as energetic, active, responsibility-seeking and refusing to give up, even though in acute pain. The ulcerative colitis patient, on the other hand, tended to give up readily when faced with a difficult conflict or a frustrating life situation.

Daniels, a psychoanalytically trained psychiatrist inspired by Murray's work, expressed early interest in ulcerative colitis. His first cases included 25 patients seen from 1930 to 1940 at the Presbyterian Hospital in New York.[5] These were not purely random cases, since most had been referred by internists for psychiatric consultation. Eight showed a pathological attachment to a close relative, and in six the death of this person was of paramount importance to the onset of the disease. Indecision about marriage was marked in two unmarried members of the group; in two others, engagement and marriage were the causes of the first attack. In three cases, the first symptoms were associated with having a child.

In two early papers, Daniels described two other cases, the first of which might have been handled by an internist with an interest in emotional factors, the second of which needed the attention of a trained psychiatrist.[6, 7] These cases from the original series are discussed at some length in Chapter 6. They illustrate emotional factors and precipitating attacks as well as the general features of the psychotherapy offered in those early years. The patients had a follow-up of more than 30 years. The second case needed not only experienced psychiatric treatment but also the services of a well-equipped social service department for ancillary assistance. In a footnote to that case, Daniels contrasted the personalities of spastic colitis patients to those of ulcerative colitis patients, and he noted that the latter have a more narcissistic character organization in which psychotic trends predominate over neurotic ones.

Daniels' repeated observation that depression and psychosis play crucial roles in the prognosis for ulcerative colitis was a pioneering contribution to our understanding of the psychogenic factors in the illness and has stood the test of time.

LATER CONTRIBUTIONS

Groen's work with ulcerative colitis began, and was reported, later than that of Murray, Sullivan and Daniels.[19, 20] His studies, therapy and approach closely paralleled the methods and the early findings of the others. Like Sullivan, he was an internist who, having become interested in the psychological aspects of ulcerative colitis, became a psychotherapist and an investigator of these factors.

Groen came to the psychological field to "scoff and remained to pray," as seen by his enthusiastic praise of Murray in his 1956 article.[19] He stated that he had originally looked into the question of the emotional factors in ulcerative colitis because all the medical treatment then existent had proved unsatisfactory and because he felt that the psychological claims would be easy to refute. He noted that all previous investigators who had seriously examined the importance of psychological factors had found them to be valid. He suggested that one reason for the medical man's skepticism had been "the almost unchallenged axiom of 20th century medicine that psychogenic factors can produce functional disease, but that organic disorders, characterized by morphological damage in the tissues, can be caused by organic pathogenic factors only." Murray's hypothesis about the etiology of the disease, Groen went on to say, contradicted this aspect of twentieth century medical thinking.

Groen confirmed Murray's original observation about the presence of special personality traits and attitudes in ulcerative colitis patients. These traits existed long before the patients developed the disease and seemed to predispose them to it. Investigators like Groen were repeatedly struck by the emotional immaturity, dependence, sensitivity, egocentricity and neurotic anxiety in the patients, and they had been inclined to classify most of them as rather severe cases of neurosis. From the psychiatric point of view, these patients are infantile personalities, predominantly dependent and passive, who crave affection, sympathy, admiration and protection without giving much of themselves to others. Like earlier authors, Groen contrasted the colitis victims with peptic ulcer patients. Initially emphasizing the lack of aggressiveness in his patients, he later discovered that inwardly they were full of resentment and aggression that they were afraid, however, to express.

Groen also noted the connection of acute emotional experiences to the onset of the disease. He believed that the majority of patients were not prepared to accept even the possibility of a relationship existing between such events and their illness. This is of special importance to the nonpsychiatrically oriented physician who might otherwise too readily accept his patients' denial of such a precipitative connection. Groen's therapy heavily relied on the supportive aspect of the patient's tie to the psychotherapist.

Erich Lindemann's work, which began in the 1930's at the Massachusetts General Hospital, corroborated the findings of Murray, Daniels and Groen. Loss of security, especially the loss of a person of emotional significance, frequently preceded the onset of illness.[26, 28] In 56 of the 87 patients followed, the loss was due to the death of the person of key significance. Rejection or disillusionment with a relationship produced a similar effect. Apparently the important factor was a suddenly decreased intensity of interaction.

Lindemann believed that his patients suffered from an acute grief reaction that was repressed, thus preventing the normal completion of the mourning process. Their morbid grief expressed itself in a sense of emptiness, in excessive hostility to any newcomer and in feelings of loss of identity similar to states of depersonalization; at times they developed morbid somatic delusions similar to those in melancholia. He was so impressed with the frequency of symptoms of unexpressed grief in acute cases of ulcerative colitis that he began an extensive study of the symptomatology and the management of acute grief.[27]

Lindemann and his collaborators claimed that, in the acute phases of ulcerative colitis, attempts at exploration by the usual psychiatric technique of reconstruction of the life history were followed by stimulation of primitive fantasies and behavior.[26] Efforts during this period to get the patient to face and ventilate his grief tended instead to precipitate bizarre reactions. They found that the patient at this stage reacted negatively to any effort by the therapist to establish direct emotional involvement with him or her. They recommended, therefore, that early contacts be brief, thus not permitting regressive tendencies, hostile feelings or affectionate attachments to develop.

On the other hand, this group tried to use a limited system of "psychological replacement therapy." After obtaining sufficient data and determining who the key figure in the patient's life was and the function that he or she performed, they utilized the psychiatrist or another available figure as a temporary replacement and encouraged identification with that surrogate. Thus, in one case cited, the psychiatrist urged the patient to read the same books he was reading and to discuss them; he introduced the patient to people on the ward to enlarge the degree of social interaction and persuaded the patient to learn typewriting because the psychiatrist had had difficulty with it. Nurses and other patients were also utilized as parental surrogates. In effect, regression was encouraged not for primitive infant-like gratification but to foster new ways of thinking and acting through imitation and identification with a stronger model. After successful psychological replacement, psychotherapy could proceed to deal with deeper issues, such as the unexpressed grief, in order to help the patient complete his or her mourning process.

The Massachusetts General Hospital group seems to have launched the so-called "anaclitic treatment" of ulcerative colitis in an attempt to deal with a particularly stubborn case in a patient who had made no progress over a five-year period under the more conventional forms of psychotherapy. Anaclitic therapy aroused considerable controversy. It received a more thorough trial by Margolin, with dubious results reported in a follow-up by Weinstock.

In citing this case, Cobb stated that after the departure of an earlier therapist, the patient refused to accept his replacement.[4] He required large doses of meperidine hydrochloride (Demerol) for the pain from an infected rectal fistula, and he also was dependent upon barbiturates. The expedient devised was to indulge him in all his desires, even to the point of increasing the doses of medication. Under this "anaclitic" regimen, he quickly developed a "relationship" with the physician. He ate voraciously and consumed large amounts of alcohol. Unfortunately, he also developed hallucinations and behaved like a deteriorating schizophrenic. At one point, he called for the psychiatrist in the middle of the night and requested milk, which he was given. Subsequently it was offered to him in a bottle whenever his infection was dressed. He soon needed no alcohol for three months. His spirits improved, the hallucinations and the delusions did not recur, and after a year he appeared progressively better integrated and talked about the "miracle" treatment. He was still well in a later follow-up.[42]

A large-scale trial of anaclitic therapy was carried out at the Mt. Sinai Hospital in New York, under the direction of Sidney Margolin.[29, 30] He advocated "superficial psychotherapy," described as "a common-sense approach by means of kindness, tolerance, indulgence, allaying of anxiety by any available trial-and-error means: demonstrative friendliness and reassurance, deliberate omniscient and omnipotent behavior by the doctor for the purpose of enhancing confidence in him, total somatic care in terms of nutrition, medication, hygiene, agreeable environment, etc." The auxiliary personnel were further instructed to build up the status and the power of the therapist by clearly demonstrating that all their activities were under his direction and control.

As in the Massachusetts General Hospital experiment, anaclitic therapy encouraged profound regression. Food was prepared and provided by the therapist on demand. Areas of pain and discomfort were massaged and stroked. A period of total permissiveness was instituted. The idea was to re-enact the genetically significant conflict at the most infantile level.

Weinstock, a psychiatrist, reported a follow-up survey of hospitalized patients treated anaclitically or by other more usual techniques between 1946 and 1958.[49] In general, he found the results of this short-term therapy to be poor, and he expressed pessimism about the ultimate value of brief therapy, anaclitic or otherwise.

In a subsequent study based on a questionnaire given to members of the American Psychoanalytic Association who had treated patients with ulcerative colitis by long-term psychoanalytical therapy, Weinstock noted somewhat better results.[50] By its nature, the study was uncontrolled and somewhat impressionistic. His report was limited to 28 cases treated by 20 psychoanalysts. All the patients had been considered severely ill and had been hospitalized one or more times.

Of the 28 cases, 14 had received psychotherapy one to four times a week for 1-½ to 5 years; the rest were psychoanalyzed an average of four times weekly for the same lengths of time. The report required at least a three-year follow-up by the therapists.

According to the reports of the therapists, 11 of 14 patients in long-term psychotherapy and 10 of 14 who received intensive psychoanalysis underwent long periods of remission, of a mean duration of nine years. Poor results were largely from patients with chronic unremitting colitis who were never free of symptoms.

The most common psychiatric diagnosis was "obsessive-compulsive character disorder." Weinstock's report made no correlation between the claimed outcome and the psychiatric diagnosis, the type of treatment interventions actually used or the somatic changes, if any, independently confirmed by direct examination. Most respondents to the questionnaire optimistically claimed that psychiatric treatment was the decisive factor in preventing recurrences and in maintaining remissions.

Daniels and the Columbia-Presbyterian Ulcerative Colitis Study Group were among the first to have developed a close cooperation among gastroenterologists, psychiatrists and surgeons. Their joint interest led to the establishment in 1948 of the Ulcerative Colitis Clinic at the Presbyterian Hospital and the Vanderbilt Clinic, in which all patients were regularly evaluated by internists, surgeons and psychiatrists. Their efforts established the value of the comprehensive combined management of chronic ulcerative colitis.[8, 14, 21–24, 38]

Another significant development was the addition of supervised psychotherapy for medical patients to the program of the Psychoanalytic and Psychosomatic Clinic for Training and Research, which was established in 1945 at Columbia. This Psychosomatic Service provided continuous and comprehensive treatment for ulcerative colitis patients and many others who were referred from the clinical services of the hospital. Patients were simultaneously followed by the Ulcerative Colitis Clinic and by the Psychosomatic Service of the Columbia Psychoanalytic Clinic for Training and Research. They formed the large group that was consistently treated and followed up and that became the basis for the investigations reported here.

To our knowledge, the most comprehensive follow-up study of the immediate and long-term effects of psychotherapy for ulcerative colitis patients was the one made at the Columbia-Presbyterian Medical Center. Its results are reported in Chapters Two, Four and Five.

Grace, Wolf and Wolff, in their monograph discuss their experiences with 19 cases of ulcerative colitis.[16] Each of the patients was repeatedly interviewed for at least 12 hours, and four were interviewed for 25 hours or more. The studies extended 6 months to 2 years. It was apparent to the investigators that the onset of ulcerative colitis and each of its exacerbations often came during times of stress. The latter were not necessarily major catastrophes but were usually related to aspects of everyday life—relationships to wives, husbands, mothers-in-law or employers, or the anxieties associated with the care of a newborn infant. Many of the incidents produced feelings of rejection symbolically related to early parental rejections. Like Groen and others, these investigators found that, in all their patients at one time or another, a threatened loss of love precipitated an attack. In their view, ulcerative colitis was a stress disorder that demanded a constructive physician-patient relationship if favorable results from treatment were to be obtained.

One of the early evaluations of the use of psychotherapy by an internist was reported in 1954 from the New York Hospital by Grace, Pinsley and Wolff.[18] Thirty-four patients with ulcerative colitis were treated psychotherapeutically by one physician (Grace), whose primary emphasis was the alleviation of stress. This group was compared with a control group treated only by the usual medical methods (steroids were not mentioned). Both groups were matched for age, sex, severity of illness, age of onset and structural changes in the colon. They concluded that in the treatment of ulcerative colitis, the physician must deal with his patient's attitudes, moods and feelings, as well as with life-threatening emergencies.

Grace and Wolff, in outlining their psychotherapeutic approach to patients with ulcerative colitis, emphasized encouraging the patient to verbalize his or her complaints and difficulties and to show feelings freely without criticism from the therapist.[17] Support should be freely and warmly given, and no problem should be considered too trivial to discuss. Special consideration must be given to the patient under stress; he should be encouraged to telephone the physician when necessary. Appointments should be rescheduled if the situation requires it. Finally, it may be important to change the patient's environment in some cases.

Some of the earliest psychoanalytical views about disordered colon function were those of Alexander and others at the Chicago Institute for Psychoanalysis.[1,2] Alexander believed that the psychodynamics of patients with colon disease could best be explained in terms of infantile fantasies being attached to excremental functions. His hypotheses were derived from the early psychoanalytical theories of infantile sexuality advanced in particular by Sigmund Freud and Sandor Ferenczi. Alexander did not state whether emotional conflicts typical of ulcerative colitis differed significantly from those in other forms of recurrent or chronic diarrhea.

Alexander held that all forms of emotional stimuli that had a symbolic connection to infantile excretory (anal) fantasies could develop a specific affinity for colon functions. Essentially, he equated excretion symbolically with acts of "giving" or "withholding." In addition, Alexander emphasized that diarrhea could represent an unconscious expression of hostility. He did caution that patients might utilize the symptoms of colitis for the secondary purposes of satisfying other psychoneurotic needs that had no causal relationship to the disease itself.

Alexander's discussions of ulcerative colitis pointed up the weakness of the ego in such patients. Like other authors, he noted also that many patients had a tendency to develop paranoid trends of thought toward those who had disappointed them. Because of this serious psychiatric complication, Alexander cautioned against too rapidly uncovering repressed impulses that would overburden an already fragile ego. For many cases, he recommended superficial supportive psychotherapy, because he believed that deeply penetrating therapy might aggravate the illness or might even precipitate a psychotic episode.

At a later period, Alexander, French and Pollock wrote that a central dynamic factor in ulcerative colitis is the loss of hope when the patients face a task involving responsibility, effort and concentration.[2, 15] The authors suggested that the predisposition to hopelessness arose in early childhood when the patients were exposed to premature or excessive challenges by ambitious parents, usually by the mothers. The mother's own ambitions were transferred to the child, along with high expectations that compelled the child to perform not for realistic aims but in order to assure him or her of mother's love. A frequent consequence of such a premature fixation upon pleasing the parent through impossible achievement is a fragile ego that is subject to disintegration and paranoia; this possibly explains the not infrequent association of psychotic symptoms with severe ulcerative colitis.

An important contribution to our understanding of the psychological background of ulcerative colitis is that of George L. Engel.[9–13] An internist who was also psychoanalytically trained, Engel was influenced to some extent by Alexander's earlier simplistic theories, but he later evolved a more complex hypothesis of the etiology and the treatment of the disease.

Engel considers psychoanalytical therapy the best form of psychotherapy but does not spell out the modifications of the analytical method that may be required for ulcerative colitis. He includes complete psychoanalysis among the psychotherapies to which he refers.

According to Engel, the maximum expectations from formal psychotherapy should be explained to the patient. Remissions might still occur without therapy, but Engel believes that psychotherapy offers a greater chance of remission. He warns of disastrous consequences that may unexpectedly occur when an analysis is terminated. A relapse with bleeding may suddenly develop while the patient is in a period of mourning over the approaching loss of the analyst as the end of treatment becomes imminent. Engel therefore advises that psychoanalytical therapy not be terminated totally and absolutely. The initiation of full separation is best left to the patient. Engel considers the opportunity for a continual, though attenuated, relationship with the internist also to be vital. In effect, the patient who has had ulcerative colitis should never be discharged from therapy.

Engel advises that intensive psychotherapy be continued as long as the architecture of the bowel seems to be returning to normal, as seen on radiological and sigmoidoscopic examination. When the disease process clearly worsens and abscesses, fistulae or pseudopolyps develop, and if psychotherapy fails to bring about symptomatic improvement or cannot be carried out owing to severe physical symptoms, surgery may be indicated.

Engel warns the psychotherapist not to turn the patient over to the surgeon without maintaining contact with him and resuming therapy after the surgery. Otherwise, according to Engel, the operation may be a failure.

Engel's views are not without inherent contradictions. On the one hand, he states that "ulcerative colitis involves some type of biologic defect of the colon and that there is no evidence whatsoever that any form of psychotherapy, no matter how intensive, can basically alter or modify this defect, any more than insulin modifies the basic defect in diabetes."[13] Psychotherapy's principal contribution is, in Engel's view, the modification of the individual's basic psychological structure to render him or her less vulnerable to those situations in which the disease becomes manifest.

Engel does not explain, on the other hand, how the alteration of the patient's personality is transmitted into greater resistance to tissue breakdown in the colon. He does not adequately account for the emotional distortions so frequently found in varying degrees of severity in the ulcerative colitis patient. He also does not seriously consider the possibility that what produces or contributes to the "biologic defect" in the colon may be the same early developmental experiences that result in a permanent susceptibility to the stresses of independence and of loss of support from others.

One of Engel's observations, which has not always been confirmed by others, is that the initial physical symptom of ulcerative colitis is most often bleeding, not diarrhea. We believe it is true that bleeding frequently announces the disease. Needless hemorrhoidectomies have been performed by unsuspecting surgeons on some patients who were actually developing ulcerative colitis. In Engel's original series of 32 patients, diarrhea was the presenting symptom in 12 cases; blood in the stools was the earliest abnormality in the majority. While this proportion may vary from series to series, bleeding is a far more common signal of the illness than is generally recognized. In our own patients, we have often also found a history of constipation preceding the onset of bleeding or diarrhea, as Engel also reports.

Engel's psychosomatic hypothesis differs from Alexander's focus on diarrhea and on the symbolic meanings of the process of elimination. The disease, points out Engel, does not necessarily begin with an integrated excretory pattern of diarrhea. He is also critical of Grace and Wolff's hypothesis that the primary reaction of the colon in ulcerative colitis is its "riddance" pattern of diarrhea. Engel emphasizes that relapses begin—usually with bleeding—when patients have been forced by circumstances to assume more independence than they can manage. Engel defines their affective state at such critical junctures as one of "helplessness, hopelessness or despair and being overwhelmed, too much to cope with, too much to expect of me."

Engel believes, as we do, that the psychological disposition to ulcerative colitis originates in the symbiotic relationship to the mother, which determines the nature of all future relationships. He speculates that separation reactions are associated with a nonspecific physiological process that has no primary psychological meaning. According to him, "when separation is not or cannot be dealt with by psychologic mechanisms (as normal grief) physiological changes are initiated in the body which interfere with or disrupt other adaptive or integrative processes permitting various types of tissue breakdown, disturbances of local tissue growth, invasion of viruses or bacteria, etc." The nature of this process remains unknown. Engel's hypothesis is nonspecific and broad enough to be attractively plausible, even if unprovable at present. Although Engel does not believe that psychological processes can control somatic functions, there has recently been a renewed interest in operant conditioning, which offers clear evidence in lower animals, for the most part (although some human subjects have been able to regulate their heart rates and their blood pressure by thought alone), that psychological (mental) activity can produce altered vascularity in chosen organs and even in parts of organs. Nevertheless, for the time being, Engel's "shotgun" hypothesis that nonspecific somatic regressive outflows occur when psychological outflows of appropriate affects are blocked or unavailable because of infantile emotional obstacles remains a helpful guide to understanding psychosomatic disorders, pending conclusive demonstration of the significance of operant conditioning on colon function.

A view strongly opposed to that of Engel and ourselves is expressed by Mendeloff and his associates.[32–34] Their large-scale studies of incidence and prevalence were not, according to the authors, intended to prove or disprove any hypotheses of etiology. They sought to compare the occurrence of demographical and socioeconomical factors and psychologically stressful experiences in patients hospitalized with irritable colon with those of patients hospitalized with ulcerative colitis and also with those of "healthy" citizens living at home.

The methodology and findings are worth describing, if only because they leave much to be desired in the view of the dynamically oriented psychiatrist.

One hundred and two patients with irritable colon; 277 patients with inflammatory bowel disease, 158 of whom suffered from ulcerative colitis and 69 of whom had Crohn's disease; and 735 healthy adults representing the general population were given lengthy home interviews. (In the case of the ill group, these were carried out after they had left the hospital.)

The interviews were conducted by "trained" lay investigators who did not know their subjects' diagnosed illnesses. These lay interviewers received two weeks of preliminary training. Different groups of interviewers replaced each other from time to time during the study.

The authors concluded that, whereas the American literature leaves the impression that ulcerative colitis occurs most often in individuals with certain striking personality characteristics, "every controlled study including this one fails to establish that these characteristics are more frequently noted in such patients than in those with other chronic gastro-intestinal disorders or even in subjects assumed to be healthy in the general population."

Although the authors recognized the fallibility of data obtained by "trained" interviewers from single interviews, their emphatically stated conclusion must appear surprisingly naive to a psychiatrist. In any case, a full and meaningful self-exposure by the patient or by the healthy subject almost never occurs until a trusting relationship with a therapist *who wants to help* has been established. This kind of working relationship between patients with lower bowel disorders, especially those with ulcerative colitis, and a psychiatric investigator may require weeks and even months to develop; the patient must slowly develop trust in the therapist until a true alliance dedicated to overcoming the illness has formed between them. To suggest that a barely trained interviewer can walk in on a stranger and, without any purpose but his hired "curiosity," elicit a full disclosure of that unknown person's personal feelings, thoughts and behaviors, tries any thoughtful physician's credulity. If the sheer weight of numbers and the pseudo-objectivity of patient anonymity in the work of Mendeloff and associates had not impressed some gastroenterologists, this type of "research" could be simply dismissed as poorly conceived, in that by its design it produces the expectation of the authors. For a psychiatrist, there is one telling piece of evidence in the findings that invalidates the conclusions drawn by the authors. After interviewing a total of 1114 persons, the authors could not cite any significant personality differences that distinguished the ill from the well; everyone ended up with similar characteristics. The only reasonable conclusion that can be drawn is that everyone wants to appear "normal"; an individual needs a strong motivation to be really truthful about his or her idiosyncrasies and personality defects—a factor these interviewers could not possibly supply, even assuming they could correctly identify those defects.

ULCERATIVE COLITIS VS. GRANULOMATOUS COLITIS (CROHN'S DISEASE)

In recent years, granulomatous disease of the colon has been distinguished from ulcerative colitis. We have presented some tentative findings about the results of treatment for both types of colitis (see Chapter Two). As of this writing, the relative treatability of each group of patients is not yet possible to determine clearly.

E. P. McKegney et al. note that Crohn's disease is more like regional enteritis in its frequency and its pathological findings on clinical and radiographical examination.[31] The term is used to describe granulomatous disease of either the large bowel or the small bowel.

The authors conclude that the patients with ulcerative colitis were not distinguishable from those with Crohn's disease. Both groups had a high incidence of emotional disturbance, of psychopathology and of significant disease onset situations. Furthermore, the study indicates that previous psychiatric findings cannot be challenged on the grounds that they did not distinguish between the two pathophysiological syndromes. The authors corroborate studies like our own that suggest a high degree of correlation between the severity of the emotional disturbance and the severity of the physical illness, "whether diagnosed Crohn's disease, regional enteritis or ulcerative colitis."

J. W. Paulley, who has treated patients with Crohn's disease for many years, wrote, "Sufferers from Crohn's disease have a personality pattern almost indistinguishable from that now increasingly accepted as a specific in ulcerative colitis and similar forms of stress are especially provocative in both diseases."[39]

In 1971, Paulley reported his experiences with 39 of 40 patients treated up to 18 years with corticosteroids, antibiotics and psychotherapy.[40] Emphasizing a subtle difference in their reactions to conflict, he stated, "The patient with Crohn's disease although sharing the ulcerative colitic's extreme aversion to quarrels or a strife-ridden environment, usually reacts differently by adopting the active role of peacemaker, whereas the colitic is outwardly more passive, more supine and sometimes querulous." Crohn's disease patients are thought of by many as "very nice people who tend to have more to say for themselves than do the ulcerative colitis subjects and are considered to be less demanding."

Paulley goes on to say that, in his experience with Crohn's disease, the commonest provocation is the "in-between situation when sandwiched between two bickering parents or a parent and sibling living in a constant atmosphere of acrimony. By refusing to agree with either side for fear of incurring their wrath, the patient unconsciously perpetuates the conflict and pays the ultimate penalty. . . . The inability or unwillingness to extricate themselves from a particular in-between situation is a sufficient therapeutic challenge but their unconscious predilection to continue the same pattern of behavior and to reconstruct comparable abrasive situations at work, in their marriages and in their children's marriages necessitates long term supervision and repeated interpretation."

ULCERATIVE COLITIS IN CHILDREN

The prevalence of and serious prognosis for ulcerative colitis of childhood are well known to pediatricians. The underlying psychological disposition is often similar to that in adults, and the grossly disturbed parent-child attachment often described by adult patients is enacted before the physician's eyes.

The earliest known study of ulcerative colitis in children was begun by William Langford at the Babies Hospital of the Columbia-Presbyterian Medical Center in the 1930s. The death of an affected 10-year-old girl on the anniversary of her father's suicide a year before led to a more careful psychiatric screening of all children with ulcerative colitis. Langford reported in 1964 on 109 cases of childhood ulcerative colitis.[25] Sixty-three of 109 patients had received some form of psychotherapy. Forty-three of the patients were followed for 15 years, through later periods of ordinary stress in adolescence, college, career, marriage and parenthood. Of this group, 23 were given psychiatric treatment, and their parents received supportive and directive counseling. The mortality rate for the untreated cases was considerably higher, and a proportionately larger number of these patients remained unimproved.

In the original group of 109 cases, a review of the records of the 63 children who had received some form of brief psychotherapy indicated that, although the basic disease process was not altered, therapy did help the children to adapt better to both physical and emotional stress and to suffer less social disability. Their diarrhea was less severe and less incapacitating. Improvement was also objectively confirmed by proctoscopic examination. The patients considered themselves much improved, unlike the children who had not received psychiatric treatment.

Langford reported the exaggerated tendency of the patients to regress in the hospital. He found that early ambulation reduced the regressive trend but increased the considerable hostility of his young patients. Langford commented on the marked difficulty these children had in accepting their own hostile impulses. Their colitis was frequently triggered, as in many adult victims, by a real or an imagined separation from a parent, usually the mother. Among older children, Langford found that 40 per cent of the exacerbations of the disease were directly related to anxiety about school and promotions.

Mohr and his associates studied six children with ulcerative colitis who were placed in a special ward where a multi-faceted treatment was attempted.[35] The children were given individual therapy, the family constellation as it related to the child's illness was fully studied, and one or both parents were given help, if required. The ages of the patients varied from 7 to 11 years.

All the mothers of the patients had experienced a lack of warmth and care from their own mothers, who were characterized as cold, severe, dominating and unaffectionate. They remained in a consistently hostile yet dependent relationship with their mothers, and although determined to do a better job of child-rearing, they lacked the formative experience of being mothered in their own childhood and so failed to develop effective patterns of mothering. Mohr found further that at the birth of the patient some event, either in her external life or directly relating to the pregnancy, made the mother less able to fulfill her maternal role. The father's relation to the illness, according to Mohr, was secondary to the mother's, but the mothers gave the impression that the fathers were also incapable of filling their parental role.

The limited capacity of the parents of the patients to meet their children's needs was repeatedly emphasized by the Mohr study. Children suffering from ulcerative colitis feel threatened because they anticipate being overwhelmed by demands that overtax their capacities. The conviction that mother will not fulfill their needs goes back to infancy and to her inability during the postpartum period to respond with comfort, acceptance and security. Anxiety evoked by the mother's failure to respond is later expressed in fantasies about the incompetent and destructive nature of the mother and about the dangerous and poisonous nature of the food provided by her. This apprehension may be extended to all persons and situations involved in the child's care.

The investigators found the basic psychological factors operating in the child suffering from ulcerative colitis to be consistent with the reconstructions made from the study of adults. Mohr and his associates further stated that the disorder in the early mother-child symbiosis that is associated with psychoses of childhood also contributes to ulcerative colitis.

Prugh has provided a penetrating discussion of ulcerative colitis in children from observations made at the Children's Hospital Center in Boston.[41] The children studied and treated were between the ages of 6 and 16 years. Prugh found an emotional component in a large proportion of the cases. The nuclear conflict that he suggested was the child's intense desire to be loved, versus his or her unacceptable and unexpressed feelings of anger and resentment toward the parents, who showed inconsistent and often confused responses to their child.

Precipitating events could generally be identified; they might range from the death of a parent to something as trivial as changes in the sleeping arrangement in the home. They resulted in a sweeping loss of emotional security and unacceptable guilt-producing anger toward the authority figures, usually the parents. In one case, the disease appeared following the removal of the child from the mother's bed when the father returned from the Army. The taboo against anger was frequently due to the parents' repressive attitudes toward the expression of such feelings.

Melitta Sperling, who began treating children with ulcerative colitis in 1942, later reported on her experience with six cases. From these six cases she branched out into treatment of adolescents and adults and over the years amassed a considerable literature describing her theories.[43–45] In an early account, she illustrated her direct psychoanalytical approach.[21] She strove to remove the child from the hospital as soon as possible but encountered difficulties in keeping the child at home because of the mother's need to be rid of it. In her early contacts with children in the hospital ward, she ingratiated herself by promoting concessions and by establishing herself as the child's ally. She described what she termed the "working through" of the child's aggression and the self-destructive reaction it produced in the child—bloody diarrhea. Sperling considered the typical symptom of ulcerative colitis to be bloody diarrhea, differentiating it somatically and psychologically from other forms of diarrhea. She stated, "One gains the impression that the amount of bleeding can be determined by the individual child," and she was convinced that the quantity of blood was directly proportional to the intensity of the unconscious rage present. She found many similarities to melancholia, such as the hostile identification and incorporation of the maternal object. The author offered the problematical hypothesis that "the destruction and elimination of the object through the mucosa of the colon (bleeding) would seem to be the specific mechanism of ulcerative colitis." Sperling classified ulcerative colitis as an organ neurosis with pregenital conversion symptoms. The anorexia, vomiting, abdominal pain, diarrhea and bleeding represented the expression of and defenses against the aggressive incorporation of the object causing frustration.

Sperling insisted not only that patients should be kept out of the hospital, but also that they should avoid medication and be kept as much as possible away from the internist. She believed that so-called supportive treatment prevents the patients from facing up to their symptoms and, even more important, that it tends to split the transference attachment to the therapist. The most important aim to her was the maintenance of a "non-contaminated transference"; otherwise there would be no real therapeutic alliance with the healthy parts of the patient's personality. For this reason, sharing the patient with other specialists is dangerous, because it "splits, dilutes and contaminates the transference"; it also serves as an excuse for the patient's resistance, in that it assigns the control of symptoms to others instead of encouraging the patient to accept personal responsibility for them.

Sperling advocated direct psychoanalytical interventions, with deep interpretations of unconscious motivations. She claimed that in acute cases this approach had been a life saver.[25] In such cases of "psychosomatic suicide," interpretation of the unconscious self-destructive impulses worked like a kind of psychological shock therapy. The therapy was given while the patient was in the hospital. It was not continued but was used only as a life-saving measure and as an introduction to the need for subsequent treatment. Sperling was convinced that only through unadulterated psychoanalytical treatment could there be a cure.

The validity and the wisdom of Sperling's extreme position have been questioned by both psychoanalysts and internists. At a 1967 Panel of the American Psychoanalytic Association, Karush voiced his doubts about the soundness of Sperling's methods and approach. He was critical of her insistence that medication, special diets and other medical procedures be totally suspended to insure that positive results could be attributed to nothing but "psychoanalytic" intervention. Obviously, such a vigorous stand would be impossible to enforce for hospitalized patients and, at the very least, difficult to control in ambulatory cases. Furthermore, Karush suggested, the strict abstinence from medication might introduce a subtle statistical distortion. Any patient who did take medical advice might understandably be excluded from the statistics on "psychoanalytic cures," thus minimizing the likelihood that all reports of failures would be made. For extremely ill ulcerative colitis patients, the ethical issue in withholding steroids, which could spare them from radical surgery or even from death, is open to serious question.

Karush also disputed Sperling's description of the nature of the transference in her cases, which he believed was created and excessively encouraged by her open assumption of magical powers.* By making the patient and the family totally adhere to her prohibition of medical supervision, she created an illusory image of the analyst in which he or she was given extraordinary powers of magical omnipotence in the patient's and the parents' eyes. He questioned how such a profoundly regressive transference could ever be properly modified later, as required by the minimal standards of a truly psychoanalytical therapy. Karush agreed that patients can be greatly helped by Sperling's methods, especially during acute episodes. He indicated that experience over a long period

*American Psychoanalytic Association Workshop, Boston, 1968.

of therapy and follow-up has repeatedly shown that many such "analytic" cures turn out to have been temporary "transference" cures. The conviction that the analyst is a grandiose extension of the patient usually cannot be worked through in the analysis without precipitating a depressive and paranoid reaction accompanied by a physical relapse. Sperling's type of therapy, whatever one chooses to call it, may be extremely valuable for those who are psychologically and somatically ill, but the patient who benefits from it will need, as Engel has emphasized, a permanent "life-line" to the therapist.

In that same panel discussion, Karush expressed puzzlement at the absence of failures in the Sperling group's reports. He stated, "We have had some extraordinary successes, but we have had failures. These failures we have laid to our therapeutic inadequacy and not upon the patient or his family. Our therapeutic failures not surprisingly have helped us understand the multiple causes of the disease at least as much as have our successes."

References

1. Alexander, F. Psychosomatic Medicine. W. W. Norton and Co., Inc., New York, 1950.
2. Alexander, F., French, T., and Pollack, G. H. Psychosomatic Specificity, Vol. I. The University of Chicago Press, Chicago, Ill., 1968.
3. Brown, W. T., Preu, W. P., and Sullivan, A. J. Ulcerative colitis and the personality. Am. J. Psychiatry 95:407, 1938.
4. Cobb, S. Anaclitic treatment of a patient with ulcerative colitis. J. A. M. A. *4*:731, 1953.
5. Daniels, G. E. Psychiatric aspects of ulcerative colitis. N. Engl. J. Med. *226*:178, 1942.
6. Daniels, G. E. Practical aspects of psychiatric management in psychosomatic problems. N. Y. State J. Med. *41*:1727, 1941.
7. Daniels, G. E. Treatment of a case of ulcerative colitis associated with hysterical depressions. Psychosom. Med. *2*:276, 1940.
8. Daniels, G. E., et al. Three decades in the observation and treatment of ulcerative colitis. Psychosom. Med. *24*:85, 1962.
9. Engel, G. L. Studies of ulcerative colitis; clinical data bearing on nature of somatic process. Psychosom. Med. *16*:496, 1954.
10. Engel, G. L. Studies of ulcerative colitis; nature of somatic processes and adequacy of psychosomatic hypotheses. Am. J. Med. *16*:416, 1954.
11. Engel, G. L. Studies of ulcerative colitis; nature of psychologic processes. Am. J. Med. *19*:231, 1955.
12. Engel, G. L. Studies of ulcerative colitis; significance of headaches. Psychosom. Med. *18*:334, 1956.
13. Engel, G. L. Studies of ulcerative colitis. V. Psychological aspects and their implications for treatment. Am. J. Dig. Dis. *3*:315, 1958.
14. Flood, C. A., Lepore, M. J., Hiatt, R. B., and Karush, A. Prognosis in chronic ulcerative colitis. J. Chronic Dis. *4*:267, 1956.
15. French, T. M., and Wheeler, D. R. Hope and Repudiation of Hope in Psychoanalytic Therapy. *In* New Perspectives in Psychoanalysis, Sandor Rado Lectures 1957–1963. Daniels, G. E., ed. Grune and Stratton, Inc., New York, 1965.
16. Grace, W. J., Wolf, S., and Wolff, H. The Human Colon. Paul B. Hoeber, Inc. New York, 1951.
17. Grace, W. J., and Wolff, H. G. Treatment of ulcerative colitis. J.A.M.A. *146*:981, 1951.
18. Grace, W. J., Pinsley, R. H., and Wolff, H. Treatment of ulcerative colitis. Gastroenterology *26*:402, 1954.

19. Groen, J., and van der Valk, J. M. Psychosomatic aspects of ulcerative colitis. Gastroenterologia *86*:591, 1956.
20. Groen, J., and Bastiaans, J. Studies on ulcerative colitis: Personality structure, emotional conflict, situations and effects of psychotherapy. *In* Modern Trends in Psychosomatic Medicine. Butterworth and Co., Ltd., London, 1955, p. 242.
21. Karush, A., and Daniels, G. E. Ulcerative colitis: Psychoanalyses of two cases. Psychosom. Med. *15*:140, 1953.
22. Karush, A., Daniels, G. E., O'Connor, J. F., and Stern, L. O. The response to psychotherapy in chronic ulcerative colitis. I. Pretreatment factors. Psychosom. Med. *30*:255, 1968.
23. Karush, A., Daniels, G. E., O'Connor, J. F., and Stern, L. O. The response to psychotherapy in chronic ulcerative colitis. II. Factors arising from the therapeutic situation. Psychosom. Med. *31*:201, 1969.
24. Karush, A., Hiatt, R. B., and Daniels, G. E. Psychophysiological correlations in ulcerative colitis. Psychosom. Med. *17*:36, 1955.
25. Langford, W. S. The psychological aspects of ulcerative colitis. Clin. Proc. Child. Hosp. (Wash.) *20*:89, 1964.
26. Lindemann, E. Modifications in the course of ulcerative colitis in relationship to changes in life situations and reaction patterns. Proc. Assoc. Res. Nerv. Ment. Dis. *29*:706, 1949.
27. Lindemann, E. Symptomatology and management of acute grief. Am. J. Psychiatry *101*:141, 1944.
28. Lindemann, E. Psychiatric problems in conservative treatment of ulcerative colitis. Arch. Neurol. *53*:322, 1945.
29. Margolin, S. G. Panel on psychotherapy in medical and surgical hospital. Bull. Am. Psychoanal. Assoc. *8*:177, 1952.
30. Margolin, S. G. The Anaclitic Factor in the Practice of Medicine, Current Psychiatric Therapies, Vol. II, Part III. Grune & Stratton, New York, 1962.
31. McKegney, F. P., Gordon, R. O., and Levine, S. M. A psychosomatic comparison of patients with ulcerative colitis and Crohn's disease. Psychosom. Med. *32*:153, 1970.
32. Mendeloff, A. I., Mark, M., Siegel, C. I., and Lilienfield, A. Illness experience and life stresses in patients with irritable colon and with ulcerative colitis. N. Engl. J. Med. *282*:14, 1970.
33. Mark, M., Mendeloff, A. I., Siegel, C. I., et al. An epidemiological study of ulcerative colitis and regional enteritis among adults in Baltimore. I. Hospital incidence and prevalence, 1960 to 1963. Gastroenterology *53*:198, 1967.
34. Mark, M., Mendeloff, A. I., Siegel, C. I., et al. An epidemiological study of ulcerative colitis and regional enteritis among adults in Baltimore. II. Social and demographic factors. Gastroenterology *56*:847, 1969.
35. Mohr, G. S., Josselyn, I. M., Spurlock, J., and Barron, S. H. Studies in ulcerative colitis. Am. J. Psychiatry. *114*:1067, 1958.
36. Murray, C. D. Psychogenic factors in the etiology of ulcerative colitis and bloody diarrhea. Am. J. Med. Sci. *180*:239, 1930.
37. Murray, C. D. A brief psychological analysis of a patient with ulcerative colitis. J. Nerv. Ment. Dis. *72*:617, 1930.
38. O'Connor, J. F., Daniels, G. E., Flood, C., Karush, A., Moses, L., and Stern, L. C. An evaluation of the effectiveness of psychotherapy in the treatment of ulcerative colitis. Ann. Intern. Med. *60*:587, 1964.
39. Paulley, J. W. Crohn's disease. Lancet *2*:959, 1958.
40. Paulley, J. W. Crohn's disease. Psychother. Psychosom. *19*:111, 1971.
41. Prugh, D. G. Variations in attitudes, behavior and feeling states as exhibited in play of children during modification in the course of ulcerative colitis. Assoc. Res. Nerv. Ment. Dis. Life Stress *29*:692, 1949.
42. Sifneos, P. E. Ascent from Chaos, A Psychosomatic Case Study. Harvard University Press, Cambridge, Mass., 1964.
43. Sperling, M. Psychoanalytic study of ulcerative colitis in children. Psychoanal. Q. *15*:3, 1946.
44. Sperling, M. Psychiatric aspects of ulcerative colitis. N. Y. State J. Med. *59*:3801, 1959.
45. Sperling, M. The psychoanalytic treatment of ulcerative colitis. Int. J. Psychoanal. *38*(Part 5):341, 1957.

46. American Psychoanalytic Assoc. Panel on Ulcerative Colitis, Dec. 12, 1969.
47. Sullivan, A. J., and Chandler, C. A. Ulcerative colitis of psychogenic origin: A report of six cases. Yale J. Biol. Med. 4:779, 1932.
48. Sullivan, A. J. Psychogenic factors in ulcerative colitis Am. J. Dig. Dis. Nutr. 2:651, 1935.
49. Weinstock, H. L. Hospital psychotherapy in severe ulcerative colitis: Its ineffectiveness in preventing surgical measures and recurrences. Arch. Gen. Psychiatry 4:509, 1961.
50. Weinstock, H. I. Successful treatment of ulcerative colitis by psychoanalysts: A survey of 28 cases with follow-up. J. Psychosom. Res. 6:243, 1962.

Chapter Four

PSYCHODYNAMIC PREDISPOSITION TO CHRONIC ULCERATIVE COLITIS

Pioneering hypotheses about the personality structure, the emotional conflicts and the mental health of persons suffering from chronic ulcerative colitis have provided significant and lasting clarifications of the psychosomatic aspects of the disease.[3–7, 17, 19, 20, 23–25] They have unfortunately lacked sufficient scope and the developmental depth needed to refine and improve our psychotherapeutic approaches. Many years of observing and treating ulcerative colitis patients have helped to crystallize the psychodynamics of the illness and the different techniques of psychotherapy presented in this and the next chapter.[9, 11, 12, 14, 15, 18] We believe they make possible a more comprehensive view both of the psychological predisposing factors in ulcerative colitis and of the psychotherapeutic processes encountered in its treatment.

Simply stated, the psychological susceptibility to ulcerative colitis begins with the disruption and distortion of the relationship to the parents and to other significant persons as early as the second year of life. During this troubled infantile and childhood development, there emerge the exaggerated emotional states, the egocentric personalities, the internal conflicts about dependence upon others and the ineffective ways of coping with the ordinary stresses of living that characterize those with ulcerative colitis. Furthermore, the peculiar nature and the prolonged duration of their early attachments to parental figures hinder those fated to develop severe colitis from establishing a clear sense of their separate identity without experiencing anxiety or depression.* This explains in large part the relatively high incidence in ulcerative colitis patients of schizophrenia and of psychotic depressive and borderline types of psychopathology, which also show a similar incomplete differentiation of one's self from others.

---

*Psychoanalysts group all persons upon whom another individual depends, either emotionally or to gratify his basic needs, under the term *objects;* that is, they are objects of needs and inner desires.

The object relationship approach to assessing predisposition to the disease was developed during a follow-up study of the responses to psychotherapy of 30 patients with moderate to severe chronic ulcerative colitis.[14, 15, 21, 22] All the patients had severe enough psychopathology in addition to their colon disease to warrant psychiatric treatment. They therefore represented a special category of severity of illness, both somatic and psychiatric. It is true, of course, that there exist colitis patients with milder somatic disease. Whether the addition of psychotherapy to the comprehensive treatment program is advisable in such cases depends upon the presence of personality traits that are functionally disruptive enough to compel the patient to acknowledge their existence and to accept help in changing them.

Seven of the 30 patients were treated intensively for two or more years, 20 for 9 to 12 months and three for four to six months. The average time between the end of psychotherapy and the follow-up evaluation of both somatic changes and psychological changes was 5.8 years.

Three rating scales provided a basis for comparison of physical and psychological improvement. Severity of symptoms and extent of observable change in the colon were measured on a scale developed by Flood (see Chapter One).[8] Behavioral changes were rated on a scale described by Klein and by a procedure that scored a composite of personality functions that reflect ego strength.[13, 16] To these ratings were added the psychodynamic evaluations by the original therapist and by the psychiatrist who conducted the follow-up examination. Psychodynamic inferences about unconscious mental processes were drawn from the descriptions of the patients' behavior during treatment. Overt behavioral changes generally reflected a recognizably improved adjustment to life. Psychostructural change, inferred from different kinds of evidence, went

TABLE 4–1 Incidence and Degree of Improvement After Psychotherapy

	SOMATIC CHANGE	BEHAVIORAL ADJUSTMENT CHANGE	PSYCHOSTRUCTURAL CHANGE
Marked improvement	8	8*	2†
Mild to moderate improvement	12	15	10
No improvement	10	7‡	18
Total	30	30	30

*Six had no colon disease at follow-up.

†One had no colon disease at follow-up. The other had shown moderate improvement but suffered a surgical "accident" during repair of a rectovaginal fistula that could not be corrected without a total colectomy. Both patients had more than four years of psychoanalytical treatment.

‡Six had no somatic improvement.

beyond adjustment; it implied a lasting alteration of some basic personality functions. Examples of structural modification of personality were the disappearance of pathogenic defenses such as denial, profound regression and paranoid projection; an emerging ability to respond to the needs of others with affection and love, which had been minimal or absent before treatment; the appropriate control of aggression, especially of outbursts of rage when frustrated; and the enjoyment of sexual gratification without guilt, infantile anxieties or inhibitions and without doubts about one's masculinity or femininity. The most sensitive indicator of maturity and of psychostructural change proved to be a shift from symbiotic dependency to stable individuation, responsibility and self-reliance in dealing with others. The ultimate test of structural personality changes was the extent to which alterations of motivated behavior, of pathogenic defense mechanisms and of infantile attitudes and needs for dependency endured through the subsequent stresses of life.

Three grades of somatic change in response to therapy were distinguished in the 30 patients at the follow-up examination (Table 4–1).* Eight patients had become free of colon disease as demonstrated by x-ray and sigmoidoscopic examination; 12 showed mild to moderate improvement; 10 were unimproved or had become worse. Psychologically, 8 had undergone marked behavioral and personality improvement; 15 showed mild to moderate improvement; 7 remained unimproved. Two patients demonstrated marked structural modification of personality for the better; 10 enjoyed mild to moderate structural improvement; 18 gave no evidence of any measurable psychostructural change.

Five distinct groups of etiological factors that affected the susceptibility to ulcerative colitis were identified. They were (1) *the psychiatric diagnosis* of the clinical form of psychopathology; (2) *the precipitating experiences of stress* that closely preceded the onset of colitis and subsequent recurrences; (3) *the predominant patterns of mental defensive processes* existing before the somatic disease began; (4) the *secondary psychological effect* upon the patient of the disease process that helped to perpetuate the illness; (5) the quality, intensity and stability of *object relationships*. A detailed discussion of each set of predisposing factors follows.

ETIOLOGICAL FACTORS IN SUSCEPTIBILITY TO COLITIS

Psychopathological Diagnosis (Table 4–2)

Patients were grouped into four diagnostic categories: personality disorder (15 cases), psychoneurosis (1 case), schizophrenia (10 cases)

*Steroids were not used to a significant extent in the comprehensive treatment of this group of patients. Their broad application came into vogue after the follow-up study began.

TABLE 4–2 Psychopathology and Outcome

		SOMATIC STATUS		PSYCHOLOGICAL STATUS			
				Improved		Unimproved	
	Number of Patients	Improved	Unimproved	*Behav.*	*Struct.*	*Behav.*	*Struct.*
Nonpsychotic	16	12*	4	12	8	4	8
Psychotic	14	8†	6	11	4	3	10
Total	30	20	10	23	12	7	18

*Seven had no evidence of colon disease at follow-up.
†One had no evidence of colon disease at follow-up.

and borderline state (4 cases). The 16 individuals with personality disorder or psychoneurosis were considered *nonpsychotic;* the 14 schizophrenic or borderline patients were termed *psychotic.* "Borderline" cases included patients with schizoid and paranoid traits and attitudes; with pan-neurotic symptoms that combined phobias, obsessions, compulsions and conversion symptoms; with hypochondriasis; and with depressive-paranoid fluctuations of mood and thought. In general, borderline patients are egocentric, occasionally behave bizarrely and seem capable only of unstable or distant object ties. It is not always easy to distinguish borderline patients from compensated schizophrenics. The borderlines have seriously disturbed personalities but as a rule do not have histories of a breakdown of ego boundaries or an inability to distinguish reality from fantasy, as shown by delusions and hallucinations. Borderline patients, in fact, show few secondary symptoms of schizophrenia, and they rarely degenerate into gross psychosis.

The correlation of the psychiatric diagnosis with the predisposition to ulcerative colitis and with the outcome of combined treatment proved a strong one and confirmed our earlier findings (see Chapters 2 and 3). All 30 patients had exhibited moderate to severe personality disorders since childhood. Although the diagnoses were not made until the patients had developed ulcerative colitis, their detailed life histories revealed the existence of neurotic or psychotic tendencies prior to the

TABLE 4–3 Precipitating Stress at Onset of Colitis and Outcome

		SOMATIC STATUS		PSYCHOLOGICAL STATUS			
				Improved		Unimproved	
	Number of Patients	Improved	Unimproved	*Behav.*	*Struct.*	*Behav.*	*Struct.*
Stress present	18	13*	5	15	10	3	8
Stress absent	12	7†	5	8	2	4	10
Total	30	20	10	23	12	7	18

*Six had no disease.
†Two had no disease.

onset of colitis. There were striking differences in the prognoses for nonpsychotic disturbances and for psychotic ones. Of the 16 *nonpsychotic* patients, 12 improved physically by the time of follow-up; 7 of these 12 had no signs of disease in the colon. On the other hand, 8 of the 14 *psychotic* patients experienced only modest improvement of colon disease, and only 1 had no sign of post-therapeutic colon disease. The illness therefore tended to be more severe and less subject to remissions in schizophrenic and borderline patients. Similar correlations were found between the psychiatric diagnosis and the extent of personality and behavioral improvement obtained under psychotherapy.

Precipitating Emotional Factors (Tables 4–3 and 4–4)

Most patients with ulcerative colitis report that a well-defined event of powerful emotional impact preceded the onset of the disease by a few days or weeks. This often seems to be the case both for first attacks and for later recurrences. Of the 30 patients in the follow-up study, 18 described such an external precipitating occurrence. The stress usually involved the loss of a significant person through death, separation, illness or simple rejection. It evoked an overwhelming sense of despair and helplessness in some. Others at first denied a conscious painful response to their experience but later acknowledged feeling a bitter sense of hopelessness, depression and resentment at the loss of the object of dependency. There also were precipitating events that only indirectly reflected an intolerance of separation from a parent or a parental surrogate. Anxiety about getting married and leaving home or about becoming pregnant (or, in men, anxiety about the pregnancy of their wives) occurred in six cases. One patient developed ulcerative colitis after her home was bombed and destroyed during World War II, although neither she nor her parents were injured. The loss of her childhood home and familiar surroundings focused attention on her vulnerability and on her defenselessness against forces beyond her or her mother's control.

We observed that nonpsychotic patients reacted more often to an

TABLE 4–4 Diagnosis and Nature of External Precipitating Stress at Onset of Ulcerative Colitis

	NUMBER OF PATIENTS	LOSS OF OBJECT	OTHER ENVIRONMENTAL STRESS
Nonpsychotic	11	8	3
Psychotic	7	4	3
Total	18	12	6

unusual external stress than did psychotics. Apparently those persons with more fragile personalities found even commonplace challenges and disappointments intolerable and distressful. While common problems in coping might not appear clearly stress producing, to more disturbed persons they nevertheless could become precipitating traumata that arouse helplessness and anxiety or hopelessness and depression. As is described in the next chapter, psychotherapy generally proved more effective sooner when both patient and therapist could identify the exciting traumatic experience that directly preceded the onset of the illness or of a subsequent attack.

Character Traits, Conflicts and Defense Mechanisms

For many years, ulcerative colitis patients have been described as persons who quickly collapse in the face of stress. A good many patients do give this impression, but the label does not accurately fit most colitis sufferers. Whether one gives up in a particular situation depends upon the connection between the stress and the patient's infantile wish to control the behavior of a particular person (object)—in other words, between the stress and the patient's confidence in his magical power to determine the conditions of his dependency. That attitude reflects the dynamic core of the narcissistic personality. When control of a dependent relationship is denied him or her, such a patient tends to lapse into a depression that has strong overtones of paranoid bitterness. Even the most passive ulcerative colitis patient has grown up with fantasies of omnipotence and desires to bind selected objects of dependency to himself. Ironically, in most cases such fantasies become apparent once illness supervenes, providing the patient with an acceptable excuse to demand service and attention openly.

It is by no means uncommon for a hospital's medical staff to tolerate and even strongly empathize with the passive, undemanding patient who never musters up any overt aggression. Let that patient begin to complain and demand more special attention and personal care, however, and both nurses and doctors recoil and resist the nagging insistence upon their constant availability and service. Since the patient may indeed be suffering severely, the attending staff's guilt may simultaneously be aroused. Unfortunately, guilt does not excite love; more often than not the guilt-producing patient is disliked even more, creating a vicious circle.

Despite the almost universal presence of this infantile self-centeredness both before and during the illness, ulcerative colitis patients as a group do not in our view develop defenses specific to the disease. They do repeat certain pathogenic defenses against stress that may operate simultaneously or in disorganized sequence. Each colitis patient regresses during illness or during the slow response to treatment in his or her own typical manner. The colitis sufferer has never renounced the dream of symbiotic fusion with a parent, through which he or she will feel totally safe but omnipotent. The belief in the exercise of magical powers to control events and people through dependency has never been replaced by individuated, independent and modestly realistic attitudes.

In addition to regression, a majority of patients deal defensively with certain drives and feelings by unconsciously converting aims, intents and feeling qualities into their opposites. These *reaction formations* are primarily directed against sexual drives, against aggression in general, and against rage and envy in particular. The sexual lives of many colitis patients are empty and arid. Inhibition and avoidance of sexual activity are prominent in both sexes. Impotence of some degree in men and frigidity or incomplete gratification in women are frequent. Aggression is repressed and is replaced by reaction formations, which often lead these individuals to be "peacemakers." If badly treated, they express natural indignation in the most unemotional, tepid terms. One young woman had become deeply attached during her prolonged hospital stay to a member of the medical staff. He had spent time with her almost daily for several weeks. One day he resigned from the hospital to go into military service without preparing the patient for his departure. She showed no overt feelings when his visits ceased, but her colitis became more severe. When a psychiatrist was brought in for consultation, she reported her reaction to the doctor's lack of consideration only as "surprise." This all too typical style of suppressing anger is related to a third defensive process common to ulcerative colitis patients, in which anger and hostility rebound against them as if they themselves were the aggressors. Masochistic traits become a common form of self-attack or of self-punishment. They accept physical pain as a deserved fate. Suffering guarantees that the attachment to the pain-inflictor upon whom they depend will continue.

Other defenses against aggressive impulses include denial and the displacement of their hostility to safer objects. Projection is a defense that ascribes one's own unconscious impulses to others. It is a particularly important factor in the predisposition to colitis, and it adversely affects the response to psychotherapy. Finally, in the most severely disturbed patients, withdrawal and defensive apathy may become so intense that the profound regression and the paranoid projection that are invariably also present in such cases are obscured.

The central internal conflict common to all ulcerative colitis patients thus reduces itself to an unresolved struggle between the wish to be dependent upon a parent or a parent substitute and the grandiose wish to control absolutely the feelings and attitudes of the object of dependency. When a parent reacts as if the assertion or the demands of the patient were aggressive and unacceptably destructive, repression of the impulse to control the parent generally follows. The dependence is thus protected for a while, but at the high price of constricting future psychological development. There are cases in which the opposite occurs. Instead of fearful submission, the patient may react with paranoid and sociopathological behavior, showing no regard for the needs and sensibilities of others. The shift to projection of blame and to accusation of objects of dependency seems to stem from the intensity of the feelings of omnipotence, from the narcissistic investment of the self with exceptional rights, and from a distorted sense of reality that substantially weakens the repression of inappropriate aggression. On the other hand, when the psychotic vulnerability to unaltered narcissism is moderated, the need to preserve the object of dependence results in the repression of aggression and in a heightened susceptibility to guilt for the "bad" impulse and to depression.

In our study, the most intense infantile symbiotic needs for dependency prevailed in two thirds of the patients. The remainder controlled and disguised their wishes for dependency or tried to deny them altogether by exerting a kind of compulsive independence that went beyond common sense. Thirteen patients were depressed, 7 were predominantly paranoid, and 10 displayed mixed and alternating depressive-paranoid reactions (Table 4–5). Although no clear correlation between the dominant mood and the outcome of psychotherapy could be made, certain differences were suggested when the nature of the depression was analyzed further. If the depression was a reaction to loss of a highly invested object or a treasured position, the treatment was more likely to succeed. When, however, the depression presented as a depressive apathy marked by withdrawal and denial of dependent needs, the prognosis was poor. The psychodynamic issues of loss-depression and depressive apathy are explored more fully later in this chapter, when the characteristic object relationships of ulcerative colitis patients are discussed.

Inner conflicts between drives and opposing counterforces other

TABLE 4–5 Predominant Mood Reactions as Related to Outcome

		SOMATIC STATUS		**PSYCHOLOGICAL STATUS**			
				Improved		**Unimproved**	
	Number of Patients	**Improved**	**Unimproved**	*Behav.*	*Struct.*	*Behav.*	*Struct.*
Depressive	13	7*	6	9	7	4	6
Paranoid	7	5†	2	7	2	—	5
Mixed	10	8‡	2	7	3	3	7
Total	30	20	10	23	12	7	18

*Five had no disease.
†One had no disease.
‡Two had no disease.

than those directly concerned with dependency are also present, although they are not specific etiological factors in ulcerative colitis. A majority of patients, for example, suffered identity disorders with distortions of their masculine-feminine self-images. Six of our patients described persistent homosexual conflicts with periods of severe homosexual anxiety.

Secondary Reactions to Colitis Symptoms (Table 4–6)

All colitis patients elaborate in fantasy even their mildest bowel symptoms to the point that they increasingly seem to threaten self-destruction. A psychical danger is thus created in which diarrhea and blood in the stools represent an exaggerated threat to life. In the dreams and fantasies of the colitis patient, danger is excited by violent emotions, which are often expressed by bowel activity and loss of sphincter control. The threatened eruption of aggression against a valued object of dependency, whether as overt hostility or as its diarrheal equivalent, intensifies feelings of helplessness and anxiety and ultimately may lead to hopelessness and depression. The clinical picture may be misinterpreted as a realistic fear of dying. What the ulcerative colitis patient fears, however, is not physical death but the loss of his favored object of dependency and of his special importance to this parental figure. In fact, one is more likely to meet a dread of radical life-saving colectomy than a fear of death from the disease. To have their bodies permanently altered, even if their lives are thereby saved, makes these individuals feel permanently inferior and repellent. Losing their body's integrity represents a castration more dreaded than death. Unconsciously, their illness or its surgical treatment signifies a kind of psychical death, since it implies permanent

TABLE 4–6 Secondary Elaboration of Colitis Symptoms and Outcome of Therapy

		SOMATIC STATUS		PSYCHOLOGICAL STATUS			
				Improved		Unimproved	
	Number of Patients	**Improved**	**Unimproved**	*Behav.*	*Struct.*	*Behav.*	*Struct.*
Repressed hostility	10	6*	4	7	5	3	5
Self-punishment	8	7‡	1	8	4	—	4
Secondary gain	6	4	2	5	2	1	4
Mixed	6	3†	3	3	1	3	5
Total	30	20	10	23	12	7	18

*Three had no disease.
†One had no disease.
‡Four had no disease.

weakness and helplessness, with loss of power to control persons to whom they are deeply attached. Conformation of the castrative significance of colectomy is found in the surprising frequency with which ileostomy patients of either sex begin to treat the stoma, which fluctuates in size, color and shape, as if it were a large penis. One woman laughingly said that she had never thought she would have had the chance to "trade" her colon for the phallus she had always envied her older brother.

The paradoxical and contradictory attitudes of ulcerative colitis patients toward helplessness and symbiotic dependency reflect the overdetermined significance that they give to "helplessness." Need and distrust are always operative and at loggerheads in ulcerative colitis patients throughout their most meaningful relationships. Persons are instruments of gratification, and to that extent they may be loved. The personal needs and feelings of such objects of love, however, seem to be of little concern. If the "instrument" fails to operate as desired, distrust quickly replaces love. In the context of this "instrumental" love, "helplessness" gains two opposed meanings. It binds the colitis patient to the "good" care-giving person who is "loved" while simultaneously producing a dreaded state of vulnerability to the very same person, who then becomes "bad," ungiving, distrusted and even hated. The presence of such contradictory reactions, which often follow one another closely, accounts for the fluctuations of mood and the unstable and capricious emotional commitments to others so commonly observed in the ulcerative colitis victim.

The importance of unconscious infantile reactions to bowel activity is often overlooked. In many chronic cases, the unconscious symbolic elaboration of the diarrhea, the bleeding and the danger of incontinence creates and maintains a high level of apprehensive tension. Some patients invalid themselves owing to the fear of leaving the vicinity of their toilet. In almost every instance, the anxiety helps to perpetuate the overactivity of the bowel and to maintain a chronic phase of the illness. It is therefore of value to reduce diarrhea by medication, if possible, and thereby relieve apprehension about their irresistible urge to defecate and about soiling themselves. "Accidents" are a source of shame and loss of self-esteem, particularly for the compulsive patient who overvalues cleanliness and self-control.

The secondary elaboration of colitis symptoms has a bearing on treatability and outcome. Colitis invites four types of symbolic reactions. There were 10 patients in our study for whom bowel activity was a favored way of discharging aggression. A typical instance was a patient who dreamed that she saw herself sitting upon the toilet, moving her bowels. As she defecated, she suddenly noticed that her mother lay dead in the bathtub next to her. She woke and rushed to the toilet with an outburst of watery stools. In another instance, a patient in an explosive fury during a therapy session shouted of her mother, "I get so mad at her, I could shit her—I mean shoot her." Eight patients perceived their diarrhea as punishment for transgressive impulses, sexual or aggressive. In their case, anger was overshadowed by a guilty need for self-punishment, which the symptoms obligingly provided. If they suffered enough they would earn forgiveness for their transgressions against the object of dependency, even if their crimes were in fantasy only. Six patients exploited their physical illness to justify demands for more and more care and attention as well as to be relieved of ordinary social obligations without shame or guilt. Those who extract so much secondary gain may succeed in making a prisoner of a parent, spouse or child, who is condemned to wait upon the patient without complaining. The caretakers surrender their freedom to come and go and to live independent lives. The fourth category was a mixed group of six cases in whom secondary gain was prominent, but in whom there was also unmistakable evidence both of inhibited hostility and rage and of the need for self-punishment. The variable effects of each of these sets of secondary responses to bowel overactivity have a distinct bearing upon responses to therapy. They are examined later in Chapter Five when the nature of the psychotherapeutic process is discussed.

Object Relationships

The nature of the emotional ties between colitis patients and others not only is a critical predisposing factor to the development of ulcerative colitis but also strongly influences the outcome of psychotherapy. Evidence of the pathogenic effects of the primary mother-child interaction and of the continuing disturbances in subsequent object attachments was demonstrated in the histories obtained during psychotherapy and at later follow-up examinations of the 30 patients.

In the course of their severe regression, ulcerative colitis patients distort the normal dependent attitudes, needs and expectations of young children. The significance of these and of other ego deficits as predisposing factors may become clearer if we briefly summarize current views of the early developing relationship to the mother and its subsequent impact upon the child's individuation. Security in his ability to cope without a parent being constantly available to "run interference" develops gradually in the growing child and ultimately becomes the central issue of self-worth in the adult. Separation from the mother without anxiety permits the emergence of adaptive capacities and leads to the acceptance of responsibility to others, which is a criterion for psychological maturity.

NORMAL DEVELOPMENT OF DEFENSES AND ATTITUDES TOWARD OTHERS

For a child to form nonpathogenic psychological defenses and appropriately mature attitudes toward others, he must successfully complete at least two adaptive tasks during the first years of life. During that time, the mental apparatus undergoes a process of "structuralization" in which basic character traits are laid down. Patterns of feeling, thinking and acting begin to take their future shape. Styles of defense against anxiety as well as characteristic ways of coping in general become better defined and self-perpetuating. The differentiation of the mental functions involved in the formation of mental "structures" leads to the establishment of the personality organization of adulthood. For example, shortly after birth the infant acts as if the expression of its needs automatically brings on their gratification. The mother's separate existence and her crucial role in the infant's life are not yet recognized. It is a stage of infantile "omnipotence" that gradually becomes shrunken and transformed into a different kind of self-regulation. The change evolves from the infant's reluctant recognition that it totally depends upon its mother for the gratification of its needs and for its security. Normally, the process of recognizing the mother as a separate being essential to the child's safety encourages the change in emphasis by which she rather than he becomes endowed with omnipotence. During this period, which begins approximately at six to eight months, the child slowly undergoes a complex transition from a symbiotic attachment to its mother to the desired phase of individuation. Ordinarily, individuation begins during the second year of life and is more or less completed by the age of four or five. The slowness of the transformation from total dependence to autonomous independence provides time for the child to form and stabilize its ideal for future attainment through identification with the loved and powerful parents. In the process, it gains a sense of its own separateness without anxiety. A sustaining sense of identity emerges—a sense of being an "I"—that helps it sort the perceptions of the outer world from inner impulses and feelings. The process of individuation makes object love possible and helps to establish firmly the ego functions involved in reality testing and in the anticipation of the future with minimal conflict and anxiety.

We suggested earlier that this complex sequence of mental changes evolves normally if at least two adaptive tasks are satisfactorily completed. The first is the development by the second year of life of a mental image or representation of the mother as an object of constancy and trustworthiness. By promptly responding to her child's needs without resentment or apathetic compliance, she helps to insure the child's lasting faith in his ability to have his needs cared for. Mother-love that is reasonably consistent and unambivalent ultimately aids the process of individuation and increases the likelihood of the emergence of an adult who can face life's stresses with the conviction, "I can do that." In other words, a conflict-free experience of being loved in this way as a child helps produce an adult with a self-sustaining sense of his own strength and worth.

The second task is for the child to master and control his physical and mental equipment as it successively matures during the "oral," "anal," "phallic" and "latency" phases of development. During the oral phase, the mouth and the skin are the dominant organs of experience, gained through feeding and through clinging to the mother. The anal phase marks the beginning of voluntary muscle control, needed for crawling, standing, walking and especially for developing sphincter control. The anal developmental phase marks the child's first efforts at separation and individuation. Attention seems to shift during the next phallic phase to the child's genitals, and early childhood masturbation becomes more deliberate. With it there is usually an intensification of interest in the parent of the opposite sex, which invites conflict and rivalry with the other parent. Latency witnesses the resolution of that conflict by identification with the rival parent and by the establishment of an internalized superego, which is a mixture of conscience, which internally polices behavior, and an ego ideal, which sets higher standards of performance for the individual. Emergence of the superego as a permanent part of the mental apparatus signals the final step toward self-regulation and a sharpened sense of social responsibility. During successive phases of development, earlier ones continue to affect behavior, but with modifications imposed by the subsequent phases. If the smooth development from one phase to the next is impeded, however, the older adaptive modes of reacting may persist unaltered, and pathogenic insoluble conflicts with the environment may occur. If the child's developmental steps meet with no serious interference or prolonged delay, he rapidly extends and adapts his first accomplishments to more and more complex matters. His new skills in problem-solving and in entering human relationships constitute a large part of the child's maturing character structure.

In those children and adults who have remained relatively fixed at the oral or anal phase, there is almost always an associated impairment in their object relationships, while their needs for dependency take on an inappropriate intensity. The different combinations of persistent infantile needs and defenses with immature dependent attachments to others determine what clinical form of psychopathology may later develop.

DEVELOPMENT OF DEFENSES AND ATTITUDES TOWARD OTHERS IN PATIENTS WITH ULCERATIVE COLITIS

The histories of adult ulcerative colitis patients demonstrate that their psychical susceptibility to psychosomatic disease results primarily from the arrested evolution of mature attachments and emotional ties to others. Out of this maladaptation flow the other distorted attitudes toward reality, the primitive emotionality, the disposition to express feelings somatically and the proneness to depression and helpless hostility typical of chronic ulcerative colitis patients. In every case, the mother (or her surrogate), who was the original object of symbiotic attachment during the first year of the patient's life, had interfered with and permanently altered her child's inherent drive for mastery over each bodily function as it successively matured. Invariably, the mother's unrelenting interferences with the normal process of separation from her control of the child's learning and decisions reduce the child's efforts at self-gratification and independent trial-and-error learning to a confusing mixture of conflicting motivations and anxieties. Instead of developing the defensive ability to guard his or her comfort or to ward off anxiety by identifying threats to security and then avoiding or neutralizing them, the child's adaptive response complies with the mother's conception of reality. Her fears, wishes or demands are unconsciously taken over by her dependent child. The need to eat, to defecate, to masturbate, to master obstacles, to compete or to cooperate may thereafter arouse opposing mental reactions in such a symbiotic individual. Natural and spontaneous impulses to act according to a prevailing need are trapped in a conflict between reality and the distorted interpretation of it imposed on the patient by the internalized image of the mother. The child who is arrested at this level of dependent attachment to the mother is fated as an adult to act as if he and his mother were one. Persistence of the state of psychological symbiosis and the child's failure to individuate and, in so doing, to give up his unconscious fantasy of "fusion" with the mother seem to predispose him to later serious psychosomatic disorders.

Data reported by others, as well as our own evidence, warrant certain hypotheses about the psychic and somatic interactions that may be involved.[5-7, 9, 18] The biological term "symbiosis," as it describes relationships among human beings, is used in a loosely metaphoric sense. It ranges in meaning from a mutually beneficial dependency during infancy to an inappropriate tie in which one partner takes over the direction of the relationship and the decision-making to such an extent that he seems to cannibalize and engulf the symbiotic partner. A symbiotic object relationship or attitude toward another person is characterized by a particular kind of behavior that seems childlike and grossly immature; when the support and the service of the needed object are withdrawn, helplessness, anxiety or depression results. The picture may be obscured by the dependent person's intense hostility and rage at the stronger symbiotic partner when his needs are not promptly satisfied according to his expectation. The dependency, however, is always close to the surface, despite outbursts of aggression and pseudo-independence.

The pathogenic effect upon a young child of the mother's emotional reactions depends on their timing and intensity and on the persistent quality of the mother's invasiveness. The functional disorder induced by the mother's intrusion as mediator and interpreter of her child's sense of reality varies according to whether its onset is during the oral, anal, phallic or latency phase of development. The earlier she interposes herself between her child and his opportunities to enjoy new experiences spontaneously with minimal interference, the more the child remains passively dependent, and the more he or she is forced to draw upon the symbiotic tie to the mother for security. The mother's compulsion to dominate each new challenge faced by the child through successive stages of development severely limits his repertoire of responses. Instead of curiosity, he feels anxiety and helplessness; instead of self-assertion, he reacts with rage to frustration or difficulty; rather than self-esteem for acts of independence, he feels guilt, as if he had defied and injured his mother and endangered his future safety. He fails to achieve age-adequate ways of displaying his emotions. Expressions of affect remain characteristic of the infantile symbiotic phase of development or the even more primitive autistic one. Emotions take on an exaggerated self-centered quality; they give no sign that another person's feelings and needs matter. More dangerously, an individual whose adaptive capacity and skills have remained so impoverished also shows a continual tendency to surrender the activation and the control of the basic body functions of eating, defecation, sleep, locomotion and self-assertion to the mother or her future surrogate. He then treats such functions as if they belonged equally to his mother rather than to himself alone, and he looks for cues from her to activate them. The expressive value of physical functions for the symbiotic child or adult seems to be limited to discharging fear or rage and to expiating guilt. In each instance, the reward for repressing his true feelings and impulses is the freedom to maintain close contact with the mother; he controls her concern and attention by the severity of his physical symptoms.

In the case of ulcerative colitis, the mother's primary interest in her child is centered upon his gastrointestinal functions, both oral and anal. She rarely enjoys quietly playful contact with her baby, but instead she expresses her maternal role by being compulsively concerned that he eat enough and excrete punctually and copiously. Once she succeeds in properly training him according to her needs, she withdraws from her child until his oral or anal functions must again be fulfilled in her compulsive way. As the anal phase develops and independent locomotive efforts by the child limit her freedom to withdraw, she tries to circumscribe his spontaneous efforts to separate. The result is a power struggle that soon involves all moves by the child toward independence, whether expressed orally, through sphincter control, or by his autonomous use of newly acquired muscle skills. When the tie to his mother threatens to be broken, the child overtly seems to give up the power struggle and, so to speak, "goes underground." His repressed conflict between holding on to his mother and at the same time ridding himself of her restraints or demands alters the purpose of his bodily functions. Instead of expressing purely biological needs, bodily functions become partly diverted to an additional use—the discharge of impulses and emotions of either hostile defiance or fearful appeasement of the mother. Natural functions thus become a two-way bridge of communication and mutual experience between the symbiotic child and the symbiotic mother, both of whom give the same functions added importance. In ulcerative colitis patients, the mother's interest is in the child's gastrointestinal functions. Through them she relates to him orally through feeding, and anally through sphincter control and an obsessive concern with cleanliness and health. The colitis victim has learned his mother's ways of showing her anxiety and "love," and he responds in kind only too well.

A facility to convert the biological function of the bowel into the psychological tie that binds mother and child together depends in part upon undetermined constitutional factors. Many children who develop ulcerative colitis at an early age are bright and precociously "tuned in" on their mother's feelings. Whether they submit to or oppose the nonverbal messages they receive, their response to reality is almost exclusively focused on the reactions of the mother. She in turn is overly preoccupied with her child's messages of self-assertion, which threaten her security. Mothers and children of this type perpetuate the existence of what is normally a short-lived symbiotic relationship. By so doing, they prolong the child's opportunity to convert gastrointestinal activity into a private symbolic language addressed to the mother. In the symbiotic relationship, the child's message is the wish to control both his mother's physical coming and going and her emotional concern. To do so, he becomes sick, helpless and dependent, as if that in fact were his mother's unconscious wish for him. Some mothers of ulcerative colitis victims openly appear to prefer their charges to remain ill and helplessly attached to them. Two such mothers became psychotically depressed when their dependent children recovered from colitis.

The conversion of the gastrointestinal tract's simple biological functions into activity with complex psychological meanings can be summarized as follows: The change in function depends upon the prolongation of the symbiotic infantile dependence upon the mother beyond the oral and early anal phases of development. Re-enactment of infantile symbiotic needs and anxieties in adulthood revives the body language of the symbiotic phase, in which intense urges and states of feelings are crudely expressed symbolically by lower bowel activity. The physical symptoms of diarrhea and bleeding proclaim the ulcerative colitis patient's helplessness in terms guaranteed to win the mother's attention and concern. At the same time, excremental overactivity may also signify rage at the mothering figure for allowing the precipitating crisis that overwhelmed the patient to occur. When the guilt for aggressive impulses cannot be neutralized by the suffering, the continuing symptoms become a form of self-punishment to which the patient seems to cling as a desperate means of reuniting with the maternal object of dependency. The patient's depression consequently grows because he cannot escape the bind in which he finds himself, caught as he now is between rage and the guilty fear of losing the dependency that can relieve him of anxiety and helplessness.

TYPES OF OBJECT ATTACHMENT

A simple system of classifying the dominant mode of object attachment was devised for our follow-up study, which applied these hypotheses about object relationships and ulcerative colitis. Patients' attitudes toward themselves and toward persons upon whom they were emotionally dependent were defined in clinical terms, as were the characteristic styles of behavior by which these attitudes were enacted. One does not need unusual psychiatric skill to use the classification effectively. It is based upon the degree to which symbiotic needs and behavior dominate relationships with objects of dependency. Patients are divided into three groups: *individuated, symbiotic* and *transitional.*

INDIVIDUATED TYPE

Individuated patients think and behave with a fair degree of independence. They have difficulty in accepting advice or guidance without automatically opposing it. On the other hand, they act as if they have every right to influence others and to control and direct those upon whom they are most dependent. While they complain of being treated inconsiderately or even cruelly, they omnipotently try to manipulate persons close to them without kindness and respect. Their self-righteousness often leads to power struggles that earn them the dislike and hostility of others. As they become aware of the failure to achieve their compulsive aims for control or to earn admiration or applause for an independent action, the importance of which they easily exaggerate, they become first enraged and then depressed. Subsequent challenges to their competence make them more and more anxious and intensify their depression. At times, individuated patients may show lability of mood to the point of appearing manic-depressive. These patients overdramatize their feelings of love and hate and are often inappropriately exhibitionistic. The majority of ulcerative colitis patients are, however, more restricted and more rigidly controlled in the outward expression of emotions. Many appear cold and intellectual. For the most part, open expressions of affection or hostility are carefully avoided, so that they appear incapable of spontaneous warm attachments. The avoidance by this group of reciprocal ties reflects their basic distrust and suspicion of the motives of others.

SYMBIOTIC TYPE

Symbiotic patients represent the other extreme. They often seem overly compliant and may act helplessly dependent upon the direction and control of others, however arbitrary and authoritarian. Nevertheless, behind the helpless facade and the withdrawal from stressful challenges lies a readiness to feel persecuted. They blame persons they depend upon for frustrations caused by their passivity and for their own shortcomings. Under adaptive pressure they become depressed and bitterly but passively resigned, and the more severely disturbed become dull and apathetic. Symbiotic patients with more labile emotionality may complain of neglect, rejection and even cruelty, but at the same time they tend to be phobic and clingingly dependent. They demand constant attention and are outspoken "injustice collectors." If their every wish is not gratified, they express their anger openly but without finding relief. They constantly remain on the lookout for objects of dependency who promise to provide care if an established source of emotional supply should fail. Constricted symbiotic patients often deny their need for attachment to anyone and cannot enjoy any close and warm relationships. They are generally suspicious and distrustful and brood over past injuries, real or imagined. When they suffer repeated failures or hurts, this group of patients often withdraws to the point of becoming apathetic and dull. They may then seem obtuse, which is really a defense against fears of being isolated and unloved and against the equally frightening danger of losing self-control, a state that invites a retaliatory attack from figures they rely upon.

TRANSITIONAL TYPE

Transitional patients probably make up the largest group. They show fluctuating symbiotic and individuated attitudes; neither predominates very long. They therefore present with admixtures of character disorders and symptomatic behavior that underscore their failure to have progressed developmentally to the phase of tolerable separation from the earlier symbiotic attachment to the parent.

TABLE 4–7 Pretherapy Attitudes Toward Object as Related to Outcome at Follow-up

		SOMATIC STATUS		PSYCHOLOGICAL STATUS			
				Improved		Unimproved	
	Number of Patients	**Improved**	**Unimproved**	*Behav.*	*Struct.*	*Behav.*	*Struct.*
Individuated	6	4*	2	5	4	1	2
Transitional	9	6*	3	7	5	2	4
Symbiotic	15	10	5	11	3	4	12
Total	30	20	10	23	12	7	18

*Four in each group had no disease.

As a group, our patients were more damaged psychologically than the general population of ulcerative colitis patients (Table 4–7). Not surprisingly, a large group of symbiotic patients was therefore included, none of whom progressed under treatment to a full and lasting remission. The level of limited personal attachment at which they functioned seemed to determine how much benefit combined medical and psychiatric treatment could provide. The connection between symbiosis and outcome is discussed more fully in the next chapter. As will be seen, however, the situation for the persistently symbiotic patients is by no means hopeless. Many can be helped and can be rescued from total invalidism with treatment tailored to their psychological limitations.

References

1. Cooper, A., Karush, A., Easser, B. R., and Swerdloff, B. The Adaptive Balance Profile and Prediction of Early Treatment Behavior. *In* Developments in Psychoanalysis at Columbia University: Proceedings. Goldman, G. S., and Shapiro, D., eds. Hafner, New York, 1966.
2. Daniels, G. E. Treatment of a case of ulcerative colitis associated with hysterical depression. Psychosom. Med. *2*:276, 1940.
3. Daniels, G. E. Psychiatric aspects of ulcerative colitis. N. Engl. J. Med. *226*:178, 1942.
4. Daniels, G. E., O'Connor, J. F., Karush, A., Moses, L., Flood, C. A., and Lepore, M. J. Three decades in the observations and treatment of ulcerative colitis. Psychosom. Med. *24*:85, 1962.
5. Engel, G. Studies of ulcerative colitis: Nature of the psychologic processes. Am. J. Med. *19*:231, 1955.
6. Engel, G. Is grief a disease? Psychosom. Med. *23*:18, 1961.
7. Engel, G. "Psychoanalytic Theory of Somatic Symptoms." Presented before the American Psychoanalytic Association, Dec. 4, 1965, New York.
8. Flood, C. A., Lepore, M. J., Hiatt, R. B., and Karush, A. Prognosis in chronic ulcerative colitis. J. Chronic Dis. *4*:267, 1956.
9. Jacobson, E. The Self and the Object World. International Universities Press, New York, 1964.
10. Karush, A. Ego Strength: An Unsolved Problem in Ego Psychology. *In* Science and Psychoanalysis, Vol. XI. Masseman, J., ed. Grune and Stratton Inc., New York, 1967.
11. Karush, A., and Daniels, G. E. Ulcerative colitis: The psychoanalyses of two cases. Psychosom. Med. *15*:140, 1953.

12. Karush, A., Hiatt, R. B., and Daniels, G. E. Psychophysiological correlations in ulcerative colitis. Psychosom. Med., *17*:36, 1955.
13. Karush, A., Easser, B. R., Cooper, A., and Swerdloff, B. The evaluation of ego strength. I. A profile of adaptive balance. J. Nerv. Ment. Dis. *139*:332, 1969.
14. Karush, A., Daniels, G. E., O'Connor, J. F., and Stern, L. O. The response to psychotherapy in chronic ulcerative colitis. I. Pretreatment factors. Psychosom. Med. *30*:255, 1968.
15. Karush, A., Daniels, G. E., O'Connor, J. F., and Stern, L. O. The response to psychotherapy in chronic ulcerative colitis. II. Factors arising from the therapeutic situation. Psychosom. Med. *31*:201, 1969.
16. Klein, H. R. A Study of Changes Occurring in Patients during and after Psychoanalytic Treatment. *In* Current Approaches to Psychoanalysis. Hoch, P., and Zubin, J., eds. Grune and Stratton, Inc., New York, 1960.
17. Lindemann, E. Symptomatology and the management of acute grief. Am. J. Psychol. *101*:141, 1944.
18. Mahler, M. On Human Symbiosis and the Vicissitudes of Individuation, Vol. I: Infantile Psychoses. International Universities Press, New York, 1968.
19. Murray, C. D. Psychologic factors in the etiology of ulcerative colitis and bloody diarrhea. Am. J. Med. Sci. *180*:239, 1930.
20. Murray, C. D. A brief psychological analysis of a patient with ulcerative colitis. J. Nerv. Ment. Dis. *72*:617, 1930.
21. O'Connor, J. F., Daniels, G. E., Flood, C. A., Karush, A., Moses, L., and Stern, L. O. An evaluation of the effectiveness of psychotherapy in the treatment of ulcerative colitis. Ann. Intern. Med. *60*:587, 1964.
22. O'Connor, J. F., Daniels, G. E., Karush, A., Flood, C. A., and Stern, L. O. Prognostic implication of psychiatric diagnosis in ulcerative colitis. Psychosom. Med. *28*:375, 1966.
23. Sullivan, A. J. Ulcerative colitis of psychogenic origin: A report of six cases. Yale J. Biol. Med. *4*:779, 1932.
24. Sullivan, A. J. Psychogenic factors in ulcerative colitis. Am. J. Dig. Dis. *2*:651, 1935.
25. Witkower, E. Personality studies. Biol. Med. J. 5:1356, 1938.

Chapter Five

THE PROCESS OF PSYCHOTHERAPY IN ULCERATIVE COLITIS

Psychotherapy may be defined as the influence of one person upon another to relieve mental suffering and to neutralize its pathogenic sources. The process can be activated by a variety of interventions. Not surprisingly, advocates of a particular therapeutic approach are prone to claim that its uniqueness or its superiority derives from the psychological theory of behavior or treatment that they champion and that their technique exemplifies.

What is indisputable is that the unpredictability of the results of treatment has occasioned the creation of an almost endless repertoire of "new" techniques. Proposed therapeutic methods include authoritarian direction, benevolent manipulation of the environment, emotional catharsis, interactional or transactional therapies, "gestalt" therapy, relationship formation, counseling, support, persuasion, behavioral therapies, family therapy, group therapy, existential therapy, dynamic psychotherapy and psychoanalysis, to name but a few of the more familiar types. *Insight* plays a highly variable role in most of these methods of treatment but is central to psychoanalysis. It is somewhat less vital to dynamic psychotherapy, although the latter is an application of psychoanalytical concepts of mental functioning.

The treatment of choice for the patients whose illness and psychodynamics have been described in Chapter Four was mainly dynamic psychotherapy. Two patients were treated by lengthy psychoanalysis. The technical emphasis in the dynamic psychotherapies varied in significant ways. Although sharp distinctions among interventions are sometimes difficult to draw, those treatments to be described were generally easily distinguishable. This was true even though it is rare for any therapy to consist of only one form of intervention. Insight therapy will occasionally and temporarily include other technical approaches, such as support, suggestion, persuasion and emotional catharsis or abreaction. It is the ultimate *aim* of the therapy that determines whether it is to be considered dynamic, psychoanalytical or otherwise. Insight remains a fundamental goal of psychoanalysis and is obtained through the appropriate use of interpretation of the patient's unconscious mental activity. Dynamic psychotherapy makes freer use of adjunctive methods in addition to interpretation than does psychoanalysis, the ultimate example of insight therapy. It is also less concerned with a thorough understanding of transference reactions than is psychoanalysis.

Psychoanalysis can be distinguished from psychotherapy in other fundamental ways. It is a long procedure and may last several years; this is not, however, its primary differentiating characteristic. Psychoanalysis tries to uncover and to interpret to the patient the nature and the origins of pathogenic mental processes and of motivating drives of which he is usually unaware. From the patient's general behavior, from his expressed fantasies, feelings and attitudes, and from his dreams, the analyst infers which unconscious processes are mainly responsible for a particular maladaptive emotional behavior, character trait or personality style. There is a heavy reliance upon the patient's *transference*, a complex mixture of illusory and inappropriate fantasies and realistic emotional attitudes toward the psychoanalyst. Transference reactions repeat and, in so doing, reveal the repressed impulses, fantasies and emotions of early childhood that may be related to ongoing psychopathological disorders. Transference also reveals pathological defense mechanisms that developed in childhood and that continue to influence behavior. It is not just a series of distorting projections and misconceptions; it also has a strong therapeutic value, because it is an integral part of an ongoing interaction with a nonjudgmental, tolerant and compassionate human being who remains as objective and truthful as possible. Out of this relationship to the analyst, both as a real person and as a screen for projections of past attitudes, the patient is given the opportunity to form a *new* attachment marked by growing trust and heightened self-esteem. In important respects, the psychoanalyst becomes a consistent and reliable model of independence and self-reliance, also providing compassion and empathy. As the patient lives through his relationship with the analyst in both its neurotic aspects and its real aspects, and as he deepens his insight into how and why he feels as he does, modifications of his personality become possible. The discovery by the psychoanalyzed patient that he has genuine choices makes his world of people less frightening, less inhibiting and less frustrating.

Dynamic psychotherapy is derived largely from psychoanalytical concepts. It aims, however, to be briefer than psychoanalysis and has more modest ambitions of altering the personality. The psychotherapist may offer interpretations of some unconscious motivational conflicts and of transference reactions that hinder improvement. His interpretive emphasis generally shifts from the conveying of emotional insights that tie past and present together to clarification, which may help patients engage in new experiences with fewer false perceptions of danger. Dynamic psychotherapy can follow two courses. It can favor the active and relatively rapid production of the patient's thoughts and feelings, which the therapist then utilizes to convey understanding, to offer suggestions and to relieve guilt or anxiety. On the other hand, the procedure may be relatively nondirective in the eliciting of material, although what is spontaneously expressed will then be used in similar ways. The goal of dynamic psychotherapy is to accelerate the processes of reorientation and readjustment so that the patient can gain a more realistic view of himself and of his environment in a relatively short time. The processes of change involved have more limited scope than in psychoanalysis and remain more closely connected to the major psychopathological disorder that brought the patient to treatment. Essentially, the patient's ego is strongly "manipulated" by the therapist's direct or indirect suggestions into manifesting the behavior that is most likely to be conflict-free and that leads to greater self-sufficiency and self-esteem.

One of the principal distinctions between the psychotherapeutic process and the psychoanalytical process arises from their difference in approach to the assimilation of insight by the patient. Psychoanalysis requires the repetitive "working through" of previously unconscious mental content. Pathogenic conflicts of early childhood are reactivated and reexperienced in the transference reactions to the analyst. These conflicts can then be brought into the patient's awareness with the help of the analyst's interpretation. Ego controls become less rigid and less inhibiting as persistent pathological defenses against anxiety-provoking conflicts are made conscious. Basic motivating drives are permitted more flexible expression, at least in thought, while the excessive criticisms of conscience and its self-punitive tendencies are moderated. All such structural changes in personality free the patient to develop, *as needed,* appropriate ways of perceiving and coping with old and new experiences. He can then become truly self-adaptive rather then being dependently guided by the therapist, however gently that controlling influence may be exerted.

Dynamic psychotherapy, like analysis, relies upon the patient's positive transference to the therapist to strengthen the effects of suggestion and to support and encourage the discharge of previously suppressed feelings. Trusting dependence upon the psychotherapist becomes the medium by which the patient is helped to give up inappropriate behavior. In dynamic psychotherapy, this positive transferential state, although a continuation of childhood attitudes toward a parent, as a rule does not itself become the subject of interpretation. Psychotherapy thus aims to strengthen the ego's weakened defenses by the *interposition of the therapist,* as an idealized powerful protector, between the patient and a threatening or demanding environment. Psychoanalysis, on the other hand, seeks to go beyond this dependency and to modify pathogenic defenses by providing insight into the patient's transferential expectations of the psychoanalyst. Analysis helps the patient to understand what he must try to change in himself and in his life situation without relying on the analyst to "run interference" for him. In psychotherapy, the therapist's role of protective ally is usually not interfered with.

We have had no direct experience in treating ulcerative colitis with what is called *behavioral therapy* or with other interactional therapies. They have come into vogue rapidly and are often opposed to the assumptions, the concepts and the aims of both psychoanalysis and briefer analytically oriented psychotherapy. Long-term follow-up reports are not available to evaluate the outcome of behavioral therapy and other interactional approaches.

Eysenck, a passionate exponent of behavioral therapy, speaks of it as the antithesis of dynamic psychotherapy and of psychoanalysis and believes it to be totally superior to either of them.[4] At the other extreme, Szasz attacks behavioral therapy and refers to it as an opposing system of belief—"one full of order, simplicity and oppression; the other of diversity, complexity and freedom. . . "[13]

Behavioral therapy generally falls into a few broad categories: counterconditioning or aversion therapy; systematic desensitization; operant conditioning, in which positive reinforcement is used; and assertiveness training, a kind of rehearsal of counteraggression. The details of these techniques and of other variations that are being introduced regularly are not relevant to this discussion, since to our knowledge they have not been specifically addressed to the special problems of chronic ulcerative colitis. The behavioral therapies require more careful and prolonged follow-up studies than they have yet received. A few behavioral therapists have begun to combine behavioral and dynamic approaches. This holds possible promise for the future, since except for the violent prejudices of extremists, the psychological theories underlying both approaches may not be mutually exclusive.[3]

Changing therapeutic styles and beliefs have recently been discussed critically by Gendlin and Rychlak in a review of research into psychotherapeutic processes during 1969.[6] They note that in contrast to the frame of reference more commonly used in previous years, "The place of intrapsychic conflicts is largely taken by interactional concepts such as roles, games, interpersonal attitudes, family systems, community and institutional structures. . . ." They report that these therapy techniques demonstrate three trends. One is a pragmatic interest in simply changing patients' behavior rather than being concerned with why they are distressed. Another tendency is to reject the idea of maladjustment being a chronic illness that needs long-term therapy. Adherents of this interactional position directly attack the deep-seated conflicts, which they view as some kind of "interaction, game or behavior pattern." Instead of providing insight, their object is to replace the older patterns with a different type of interaction, role or behavior. A third trend is to convert the therapeutic method into an instructional system. The patient is given specific steps to follow, which include instructions about relaxation, "guided imagery" and "changing the consequences," all designed to create new modes of behavior in a given situation, *regardless of the patient's ability to perceive them as appropriate models for or basic approaches to all human relationships*. The extent to which manipulative techniques like these can favorably influence the course of a chronic disease like ulcerative colitis remains unknown.

In the evaluation of the immediate and long-term effects of dynamic psychotherapy and psychoanalysis that follows, a limited selection of the most widely practiced techniques of intervention have been singled out. Our conclusions are concerned only with the therapeutic impact of *interpretation, clarification, support, suggestion, persuasion, emotional catharsis* or *abreaction*, and *environmental manipulation*.[9]

Although we shall speak of treatments as being based upon a particular mode of therapeutic intervention, few psychotherapies consist of a single method. In deciding that a technique reflects a specific style or modality, we are simply emphasizing the predominant intervention practiced in the therapeutic process. A treatment procedure considered supportive may also include emotional catharsis or interpretation of unconscious thoughts and feelings; "support," however, best describes the overall thrust of the process, the principal intent of the therapist and the kind of subjective benefit gained by the patient.

It is important to remember also that psychotherapy may tap forces that, if properly released, have the potential for positive change, regardless of the practitioner's frame of reference and why he thinks his treatment has apparently worked. All persons, despite their sophistication, cultural breadth or intellectual attainments, are suggestible. Anyone who has suffered sufficient stress to cause him to feel unable to cope may "take the attitude of the other," especially when receiving support, tolerance and understanding from that other person.[10]

Suggestibility tends to convert almost every intervention partly into a suggestion that is welcomed by the patient in need of help. Suggestion thus takes on the force of a "magical" remedy. Any influencing relationship—medical, religious, cultist or fraudulent—can therefore point to "success," usually short-lived, to justify its therapeutic value, although the subject's suggestibility alone may have been responsible. In other words, the magical suggestion that help is at hand, is omnipotent and is guaranteed to work can be conveyed by any influencing relationship in a therapeutic setting.

This complication makes the evaluation of any psychotherapeutic method difficult. It is necessary for us to identify carefully the various kinds of influence that may be legitimately exercised in a therapeutic situation and to determine which techniques best fit particular patients' needs. The ultimate criterion for a "legitimate" intervention, whether it be suggestion or otherwise, is that it not exploit the patient's dependency for the therapist's personal gain.

In every treatment, there is a critical interplay between the therapist and his patient.[1, 2, 12, 14, 16] The therapist develops feelings and attitudes of acceptance or rejection, exhibits therapeutic optimism to some extent and uses a characteristic style of intervention. On the other hand, the patient always reacts more or less overtly to his therapist's personality and operational style, to the length and the cost of the treatment, and to the specific techniques of intervention deliberately or inadvertently used by the therapist. The psychotherapeutic situation thus includes factors introduced by the therapist, by the patient, and by the nature and structure of the treatment process. The third factor includes such things as the frequency of sessions, the duration of treatment, the kind of subject matter emphasized by the therapist and the intensity with which the content is examined and interpreted. There are always variables introduced by the physical symptoms and disability caused by the disease that the psychotherapist cannot control without the cooperation of the internist and the surgeon.

FACTORS INTRODUCED BY THE THERAPIST

The aims and methods that the psychotherapist believes he pursues may, as we have said, not be entirely responsible for the outcome of the treatment. His personality, his emotional responsiveness and his style of communication, of which he may be partially unaware, often have as much impact upon the patient as his theory of psychotherapy.

In reviewing the details of the 47 psychotherapeutic treatments of our 30 ulcerative colitis patients, we could identify seven fairly distinct kinds of intervention, as well as different emotional attitudes and styles of interaction. In evaluating the effect of a given psychotherapy, one should remember that many factors play variable parts. It is difficult, therefore, to be precise about exactly what causes what to happen. Nevertheless, we have tried to find some order in the therapeutic process, which may help fit therapist to patient with more assurance and thus ultimately improve the outcome. Reasonable differences in judgment about the interplay of the factors involved are to be expected. Our conclusions were drawn as accurately and objectively as possible from the data from various treatments studied and followed-up, which we have described elsewhere.[7, 9]

Techniques of intervention will be considered first. All forms of dynamic therapy utilize these techniques, in varying combinations. Although seven modes of intervention could be identified, for purposes of comparison they can be grouped into three broad patterns: (1) *interpretations,* designed to produce three different kinds of insight; (2) *catharsis* of feelings, *support,* and *direct suggestion;* and (3) *manipulation* of the patient's environment and life situation.

Interpretation can be addressed primarily to unconscious aggressive and pleasure-seeking motivations. A second focus is on the combination of psychological defenses, character traits and resistances to change typical of each patient. Third, interpretation may deal with transference reactions occurring during treatment and with the patient's preferred kinds of interpersonal relationships, which cause him difficulties.

The ultimate goal of interpretation is insight or understanding accompanied by a sense of emotional conviction. Insight is, of course, a universal experience that can occur without therapy. It may be stimulated by a casual comment made by someone else, or by a significant association made in one's own thoughts. Insight is the deliberate *aim* of interpretation, however, because of the assumption that it makes desirable changes in behavior more certain and more lasting. In this sense, it is a sign of emotional learning. As a therapeutic effect, it occurs after a clarifying remark or a succinct statement that connects the present and past experience of the patient with his or her behavior in a causal way. The production of insight usually requires repeated interpretations of the patient's mental processes. It takes time before the assimilation of an interpretation can lead to a firm change in the patient's self-knowledge about his deeper motivations and feelings.

Interpretation does not necessarily produce insight. It may provide intellectual understanding without the affective component. Although it is not insight, understanding may help the patient to control certain forms of behavior.

As we noted earlier, interpretations generally deal with three kinds of mental content. A therapist can uncover unconscious motivating drives and emotional forces that have persisted from early childhood. He turns the patient's attention to the ongoing effects of primal urges common to all of us, but which in the normal course of development are tamed and redirected. The therapist also alerts him or her to excessive unconscious guilt that if left unaltered invites repeated physical or social self-injury as a morbid form of self-punishment. At other times, interpretation may be aimed at certain functions and activities of the ego, the mind's "organ" of adaptation. Psychological defenses that once may have served well but are now pathogenically rigid or inappropriate, as well as maladaptive character traits, are also targets of ego interpretations. Another goal of interpretation is the analysis of troubled relationships that are formed or sought with significant persons throughout the patient's life. Particular emphasis may be given to the patient's *transference* reactions to his therapist, both in psychoanalysis and in psychotherapy.

All three types of interpretation are exhaustively pursued in psychoanalysis, which aims to make conscious the origins and the forms of those mental processes responsible for current disordered behavior. In dynamic psychotherapy, interpretation is seldom as thorough and far-reaching. It may be directed in a limited way to the ongoing disturbances of behavior, or it may superficially explore any or all of the three areas just described.

Many patients with psychosomatic disease benefit substantially from a selective emphasis upon an interpretation of limited depth. A relatively small number (two of our patients) obtain more lasting relief and achieve fundamental personality changes from the far-ranging and intensive psychoanalytical approach.

Support, catharsis and *suggestion* are three technical interventions that usually occur together. They predominate in therapies for which the interpretation of unconscious mental processes is generally contraindicated and in which producing insight is secondary to maintaining the patient's dependent security in the transference relationship to his therapist. *Support* is conveyed by the physician's evident interest, by his tolerant acceptance of the patient's attitudes and limitations, by the warmth of his expression and by a genuine understanding of and empathy with the patient's feelings. A patient is supported when, on the verge of helplessness or inappropriate impulsiveness, he receives useful clarifying explanations or suggestions for coping with a stressful situation without being embarrassed or patronized. He will be especially strengthened if the therapist can counteract irrational shame or guilt by serving in effect as an auxiliary nonpunitive "superego" or conscience, temporarily neutralizing the voice of the patient's own harshly critical conscience. Since guilt-producing issues are usually minor or even imagined transgressions, there is little danger that the patient will be encouraged to indulge in antisocial behavior.

Once a trusting dependence upon his therapist's views of reality has developed, the patient becomes freer to vent emotions that he had previously suppressed. *Catharsis*, or the discharge of feelings (especially of rage), may produce dramatic symptomatic relief in ulcerative colitis, at least for a time. Intense affects may be directed at the therapist but more often will be displaced to other persons. In either case, if it is to give relief, the abreaction should receive the therapist's tacit or even explicit encouragement. The indirect suggestion to "let yourself go" is naturally embodied in supportive attitudes toward the patient. An "invitation" to reexperience repressed feelings and thoughts can be accepted if the therapist has transmitted—by attitude more than by word—his reassurance that there will be no punitive consequences. The process obviously requires care and sensitive management by the therapist to prevent irrational and uncontrollable discharges of feelings. *Direct suggestion*, as opposed to the indirect suggestion implicit in leading questions, in support and in interpretation, is generally useful only in the more infantile dependent patients. Its impact often goes beyond the immediate situation. Direct suggestion affects the patient's distorted view of reality, replacing it with that of the therapist. Direct suggestion may *seem* to sharpen the patient's understanding of his relationships to others, at least intellectually. In fact, however, he is simply encouraged to identify *imitatively* with the parentified therapist. Telling a patient what to do or to say may temporarily temper apprehensive or hostile paranoid feelings. It may often be the only way to treat a suspicious patient's persecutory anxiety and, in so doing, to ameliorate his somatic symptoms as well. Magical identification with the therapist may seem a childlike process, but it can materially ease depression in colitis patients. Direct suggestion in severe cases like these may temporarily halt a patient's regressing to the state of helplessness and despair that disabling ulcerative colitis can so easily induce. Suggestion can help him or her to give up the secondary pleasure in forcing parent surrogates to devote themselves exclusively to his or her desires. If suggestion succeeds, the patient may even recognize that living and dying are largely up to him and not his caretakers.

Manipulation of the patient's environment and life situation is a third category of intervention. Whatever form manipulation may take, it involves the interposition of the therapist between the patient and significant figures in his or her life. It occurs, for example, when the therapist meets with a parent or a spouse, talks to a teacher or intervenes with an employer to obtain some special consideration or privilege for the patient. Interposition also takes place when a therapist directly commands or forbids the patient to perform an act directed toward or against others or one that would make a major change in the patient's life for which he is psychologically unprepared. When manipulation dominates the therapeutic picture, it is of limited value; hence, it is useful only for the most helpless and regressed patients.

The outcome of therapy is correlated with the correct use of a particular approach for a particular kind of patient. When the level of object relationship (symbiotic, transitional or individuated)* at which a patient is functioning is properly matched with an appropriate therapeutic approach, the somatic and psychological results often improve dramatically.

Interpretation is best reserved for those ulcerative colitis patients who have reached the individuated stage. If used excessively for symbiotic subjects, the outcome is poor. In our study, interpretation and insight led

*Defined in Chapter Four.

to marked improvement with no evidence of disease at follow-up in the two individuated patients treated by psychoanalysis, and also in two of five transitional patients treated by dynamic psychotherapy of briefer duration. All symbiotic patients remained unimproved when interpretation was the predominant therapeutic technique and insight was the primary goal.

The triad of support, catharsis and suggestion is effective with individuated, transitional and symbiotic colitis patients, but to varying degrees. When interpretation plays a supplemental role, individuated patients respond well. Two of three patients treated by this combination of techniques were markedly improved at follow-up examination, showing no signs of disease. Transitional patients, however, are best helped by the "support triad." Two in our series were without disease after this treatment, while five of six patients were moderately improved after use of the support triad alone.[7] Symbiotic patients, as a group, did relatively poorly. There were no instances of total remission, although 12 of 19 did improve significantly. In general, catharsis seems to be more effective in individuated or transitional patients than in symbiotic patients. Support gives the best results in symbiotic individuals. Direct suggestion is moderately helpful for transitional and symbiotic patients, but it is much less effective in individuated persons.

Manipulation of the environment seems to be the least useful intervention in the long run in *all* cases. Only one symbiotic patient in our group improved somewhat when treated almost entirely by the manipulation of his life situation. Its most effective application is in *emergency* treatment of acutely and severely ill colitis patients.

It seems, therefore, that the outcome of dynamic psychotherapy depends on how well the interventions match the degree of individuation the patient has achieved. Insight therapy is most likely to succeed in patients who have a clear sense of their separate identity and who have proven capable of realistic independence. Their needs for dependency are less demanding and are not as critically important to their feelings of safety. The triad of support, catharsis and suggestion can be effective in individuated patients but is best reserved for the transitional or symbiotic patients with ulcerative colitis. Patients with the least differentiated identities, and who therefore try to "live" through symbiotic attachment to others, have the greatest difficulty in assimilating interpretations of their unconscious mental processes. In this group, change is based on more primitive mental processes, such as identification with an apparently omnipotent parental figure. Identification signifies the mental assumption by one person of the admired or envied features of another. Support and carefully chosen suggestions, both of which facilitate identification, are best suited to the therapy of the extremely symbiotic ulcerative colitis patients.

EMOTIONAL ATTITUDES OF THE THERAPIST

Another group of factors important to the outcome of psychotherapy are those that are not deliberately introduced by the therapist and are therefore less conscious and less easily controlled by him; these are the established qualities of his personality and character.[2, 16] We have found that psychotherapists may be divided into two groups. One tends to be strongly interactive and to engage in continual verbal exchanges with patients. Such active therapists overtly respond quickly to their patients' behavior and complaints and often become directive and authoritarian. Therapists in the second group are comparatively nonactive or may even be passive, and are slow to react overtly. These nonactive therapists remain quiet and soft-spoken and are often tentative and nondirective in approach and temperament. It is not that either group practices "good" or "bad" psychotherapy; rather, each shows characteristic reactions to different kinds of patients and stimulates typical transference responses in them. The attitudes, values and moral positions of a therapist and his typical ways of communicating them inevitably delimit the kind of relationship a patient is likely to develop with him.

Active therapists may intervene too quickly and thus interrupt associative trends in their patients that, if followed more gently and tolerantly, might have led to a more convincing self-understanding than is usually provided by an all-knowing therapist. Some "activist" therapists commit egregious errors because they listen badly and explain prematurely. They may ignore the patient's messages because they are preoccupied with their own pet preconceptions. There are other instances in which the overactivity of the therapist reinforces infantile passivity in a patient, totally inhibiting a spontaneous expression of anger or verbal aggression that might have helped relieve the illness. Another common problem of overactive therapists is their tendency to declaim interpretations that are superficial and impulsively delivered without adequately preparing the patient. Sometimes their interventions reflect impatience with and even irritation at a "slow" or resistive patient. In summary, overactive therapists run the risk of talking too much and listening too little as a defense against patients who make them anxious.

The relatively passive approach of nonactive therapists invites much more free association of ideas. In some patients, that freedom may create anxiety and negative attitudes toward therapy. These individuals are easily threatened by the emergence into consciousness of frightening fantasies of an aggressive or erotic nature. Nonactive therapists may also alienate certain patients because they give an impression of uninvolvement and of emotional detachment from their patients. Some "distant" therapists may, in fact, use passivity as a defense against a patient's coercive demands for dependency. A common problem among the nonactive therapists is excessive slowness and hesitancy in offering helpful interpretative or clarifying comments or in providing needed emotional support to a patient. The issue here, as in the active group, can be reduced to the optimal pairing of a particular kind of therapist with the patient who can benefit most from his therapeutic style.

We have found that while there is no overall superiority of "active" therapists over "nonactive" therapists, or vice versa, each has advantages over the other in working with specific kinds of psychopathological disorders. Moderately active therapists generally have better success with nonpsychotic patients. Nonactive therapists, if not extremely passive and unresponsive, have slightly better success with psychotic patients, and produce favorable results that last longer. Interestingly, the rare ulcerative colitis patient who is suitable for psychoanalysis tolerates nonactivity well. This individual does the best, however, with a therapist capable of exchanging his nondirective stance for firm activity during the periods of inner crisis that accompany the patient's assimilation of painful insights or during periods of unexpected stress.

Specific emotional reactions of psychotherapists can be recognized and roughly quantified during the course of a treatment. Six qualities may be observed: interest, empathy, optimism or hopefulness, proneness to quick and impulsive intervention, patience, and tolerance of a patient's hostility toward his therapist or others. Of the six, the first three—interest, empathy and hopefulness—have in our experience correlated most consistently with lasting physical and psychological improvement due to therapy. For example, when all three qualities were rated highly in a therapist, there was a 90 per cent correlation with notable somatic improvement in the patient. The presence of empathy and interest without clearly communicated optimism about the patient's chance for recovery reduced the correlation to 79 per cent. The other attitudes by themselves had much less impact upon the outcome of psychotherapy, although they still had some significance.

EMOTIONAL ATTITUDES OF THE PATIENT

Intense transference reactions tend to develop in almost every case. In fact, when they seem to be absent, results of therapy become poor. Because of transference, the therapist is treated like a parental figure, and early childhood anxieties about the dominant parent's actions are easily redirected toward the therapist.[5, 8] If the therapist cannot recognize and tolerate his patient's ambivalence, the treatment soon ends in a painful impasse, very much like that the patient experienced in childhood. It is particularly important for the patient to develop the belief that his therapist will remain a reliable object of dependency who is tolerant and noncritical regardless of the patient's provocations and infantilism.

Like the therapist's attitudes of empathy, interest and optimism, the patient's hopefulness and trust have the highest correlation with a positive outcome. Magical expectation of the therapist and hesitancy in applying the "lessons" of therapy are generally "par for the course" and occur in all colitis patients.[15] They will often display aggression in their efforts to manipulate the therapist or will become either oppositional or excessively obedient to suggestion. Not one of these reactions by itself critically affects the prognosis. One favorable quality, however, is the patient's ability to interact actively with the therapist during their sessions. There is one attitude of the patient that has a poor prognostic significance: denial, especially in the form of disavowal by a patient of the inappropriateness of his wishes and of his attitudes toward others. This is a warning that he is severely symbiotic and is unlikely to change the egocentricity that makes his relationships with others inevitably stressful.

Whether a patient remains passive seems less important than the therapist's reactions to the inactivity. Irritable impatience tends to intensify the patient's depression and his feeling of helpless anger at not being understood.

The most powerful force for somatic and psychical recovery is the combination of the patient's hopefulness and trust with the therapist's interest, empathy and optimism. Another favorable prognostic factor is the ability of the patient in treatment to change unfavorable situations in his life. Reactions to parents, school, career, marriage and parenthood are particularly sensitive barometers of adaptive strengths. We have found that patients who failed to resolve difficulties in any of these areas during or after psychotherapy had a low—22 per cent—rate of physical improvement. Favorable change by the patient in even one area raised the rate of improvement to 75 per cent, and when the patient effectively changed three of the areas of social functioning, it rose to 92 per cent.

A patient's capacity to raise the level at which he forms dependency relationships also has a strong correlation with physical recovery. We have found an improvement rate of 88 per cent among patients who could move from symbiotic attachments to more individuated and self-sufficient ones. By contrast, only 37 per cent of those who remained symbiotic after therapy experienced some improvement in their colitis. Similar differences in outcome were found between transitional individuals who could change their dependency levels and those who could not.

Among other influences upon the outcome of psychotherapy, the length of treatment has a special significance. In general, the longer the treatment, the better the results. For example, the two carefully selected patients who were treated by psychoanalysis longer than four years showed marked and lasting psychological improvement. One remained free of physical signs of colitis for more than 17 years of follow-up. The other suffered a serious surgical "accident" during repair of a rectovaginal fistula that ultimately necessitated a colectomy. Nevertheless, striking personality changes have been maintained approximately 20 years. Fifty-six per cent of patients treated one year or less improved physically, compared to an 83 per cent physical improvement rate among those treated one to three years by psychotherapy.[8,9,11]

In summary, if we properly identify the nature of the dependency attachments needed by a patient, if we pair him with the appropriate therapist, and if we select the optimal technique of psychotherapeutic intervention and continue it long enough, the prognosis for somatic and social improvement from the addition of dynamic psychotherapy to the treatment becomes significantly more favorable.

The next chapter presents illustrations of psychoanalytical therapy and of dynamic psychotherapy of the varying lengths and types used in ulcerative colitis patients.

References

1. Betz, B. J. Experiences in Research in Psychotherapy with Schizophrenic Patients. *In* Research in Psychotherapy, Vol. 2. Strupp, H. H., and Lubursky, L., eds. American Psychological Association, Washington, D. C., 1962.
2. Betz, B. J. Studies of the therapist's role in the treatment of the schizophrenic patient. Am. J. Psychiatry *123*:963, 1967.
3. Brady, J. P. Psychotherapy by a combined behavioral and dynamic approach. Compr. Psychiatry *9*:536, 1968.
4. Eysenck, H. J. Behavioral Therapy and the Neuroses. Pergamon Press, Oxford, England, 1960.
5. Freud, S. Splitting of the ego in the process of defense. Standard Edition *23*:275, 1940.
6. Gendlin, E. T. and Rychlak, J. F. Psychotherapeutic processes. Annu. Rev. Psychol. *21*:155, 1970.
7. Karush, A., and Daniels, G. E. Ulcerative colitis: The psychoanalyses of two cases. Psychosom. Med. *15*:140, 1953.
8. Karush, A., Daniels, G. E., O'Connor, J. F., and Stern, L. O. The response to psychotherapy in chronic ulcerative colitis. I. Pretreatment factors. Psychosom. Med. *30*:255, 1968.
9. Karush, A., Daniels, G. E., O'Connor, J. F., and Stern, L. O. The response to psychotherapy in chronic ulcerative colitis. II. Factors arising from the therapeutic situation. Psychosom. Med. *31*:201, 1969.
10. Mead, G. Mind, Self and Society. Univ. of Chicago Press, Chicago, Ill., 1934.
11. O'Connor, J. F., Daniels, G. E., Flood, C., Karush, A., Moses, L., and Stern, L. O. An evaluation of the effectiveness of psychotherapy in the treatment of ulcerative colitis. Ann. Intern. Med. *60*:587, 1964.
12. Pollack, I. W., and Kiev, A. Spatial orientation and psychotherapy: An experimental study of perception. J. Nerv. Ment. Dis. *137*:93, 1963.
13. Szasz, T. Behavior Therapy and Psychoanalysis. Medical Opinion and Review, New York, 1967.
14. Silverman, J. Personality trait and "perceptual style" studies of the psychotherapists of schizophrenic patients. J. Nerv. Ment. Dis. *145*:5, 1967.
15. Sperling, M. The role of pregenital conflicts and of somatic symptomatology in phobia. Read at the mid-winter meeting of the American Psychoanalytic Assoc., New York, Dec. 16, 1967.
16. Whitehorn, J. C., and Betz, B. J. Further studies of the doctor as a crucial variable in the outcome of treatment with schizophrenic patients. Am. J. Psychiatry *117*:215, 1960.

Chapter Six

CASE HISTORIES

Case One: A Psychoanalytical Therapy

The patient, a 32-year-old woman, had experienced the death of her fiance 18 months before the present hospitalization. She was referred for psychoanalysis during this in-patient treatment of an acute attack of ulcerative colitis. Because medical therapy had failed to control the disease after a few weeks, colectomy was being considered. Psychiatric intervention was seen as a "last resort" by the medical department. After the initial consultation, it was decided that intensive psychoanalysis would be tried as the treatment of preference.

Analysis began one-and-a-half years after the onset of the ulcerative colitis, which involved the distal end of the transverse colon, the descending colon and the rectum. The patient was bedridden and suffered 10 to 20 bloody stools per day.

During the first eight weeks, her psychoanalytical treatment took place in the hospital. The patient was taken to the analyst's hospital office in a wheelchair, which enabled her to sit up and face him. Appointments were arranged and faithfully kept at predetermined intervals and at stated times; she was seen for one-hour sessions four times a week. Special care was taken by the analyst to be reliable in his attendance and constant in his manner, because six months earlier, during the patient's first hospitalization, a psychiatric resident had briefly worked with her in a haphazard and frustrating way. The experience had not been good and had reinforced some of her basic conflicts. At the first analytic session, she was pale, thin and in obvious distress. She complained of bloody diarrhea, severe tenesmus and almost constant abdominal pain, was depressed and was frankly pessimistic about the future. There were poorly concealed expressions of resentment toward and complaints about her doctors, nurses, other patients and members of her family. Her faultfinding was delivered in a controlled and apparently reasonable way. The reproaches were accompanied by careful reassurances that she recognized, of course, that no one had intentionally harmed her.

The patient had grown up in a home in which reserve, self-reliance and discipline were emphasized. Her father was an intelligent, self-educated, reserved and undemonstrative man who advanced himself economically and in status through work, which often took him away from home.

The patient's mother, the dominant figure in her life, was an ambitious, controlling woman who displayed no affection toward her children and was a strict disciplinarian, quick to punish any infractions of her rules. She gave little attention or understanding to any of her children, although the patient was convinced that her mother preferred her brothers to her, the only girl. The mother was apparently a moody and disturbed woman whose outbursts of rage were unpredictable and frightening, except when her husband was home. The patient's father was her refuge from the mother. The mother was described with ill-concealed hostility and the father with idealized affection and a sense of loss, even though he had died in a tragic accident when the patient was 16 years old.

Her mother missed no opportunity to impress upon the patient that she had been an unwanted "accident" and was responsible for her mother's numerous real and hypochondriacal complaints. The mother successively developed hyperthyroidism, hypertension and finally terminal carcinoma of the rectum, during which time she became grossly paranoid, particularly about her daughter. The mother died four years before the onset of the patient's ulcerative colitis.

Competition with her siblings centered largely on gaining their father's preference and approval. She could win the struggle only through scholastic success. As an early adolescent, she cultivated a reserved and unemotional exterior; she intellectualized and rationalized her hostility at life's unfairness and tended to externalize to others the responsibility for her discomforts.

Before puberty, she had had frequent tantrums and had fought constantly with her brothers, who had made her their scapegoat. She not only lost the battles but also was usually humiliated by her mother. One of her brothers did offer some protection from the others, even though he had a long-standing chronic illness. The patient treated him as an idealized parent surrogate until his early death.

From the age of seven, she had suffered from a series of persistent illnesses that earned her the added attention and concern of her mother and father. At 16, she developed symptoms of hyperthyroidism, like the mother, and underwent a thyroidectomy. Her convalescence was slow, and during it she suffered from persistent depression.

Her father's death occurred several months after her surgery. She did not recall mourning or showing overt depression, but her mother became deeply depressed and increasingly paranoid, blaming the patient for the father's death. At times, she was told that her illness and surgery had "killed" him; at other times, that her compulsive orderliness and cleanliness had "driven him away from his home to his death"—accusations that may have been truer of the mother than of the daughter.

The mother died four years before the patient's present illness began; her vilifications of the patient, however, were taken up by some of her siblings, who called her callous, selfish and without feeling. Her helpless resentment mounted, as did her guilt and moderate depression, which lasted about a year following her mother's death. The only physical symptoms during this period were chronic constipation and periodic sinusitis.

A year before her colitis was diagnosed, she had fallen in love with a young man. He had less education than she and had no professional training (unlike the patient). Following a brief courtship they became engaged, despite the outspoken opposition of her family. He was drafted three months afterward and was killed several weeks later. Within three weeks of his death, her first clear symptoms of ulcerative colitis began—bloody diarrhea and abdominal pain. The disease was unfortunately incorrectly diagnosed and was aggravated by an unnecessary appendectomy.

As after her father's death, the patient stoically showed no grief and did not openly mourn her fiance. There was a gradual deepening of depression, however, and shortly afterward her colitis symptoms appeared. While recollecting this period of pain, she told her analyst that she now blamed her unsympathetic relatives for her unnatural restraint of emotion.

The patient's analysis seemed to move through three phases. The changing content and the emotional thrust of this patient's analysis were roughly similar to those observed in any other psychoanalysis. Rapidly improved mood changes and shifts from seemingly mature attitudes to regressed ones, of which extreme dependence upon the analyst is the most common, occur frequently, usually early in treatment.

The *first phase* of this patient's analysis was typical of the opening period of many analyses. As in this patient's therapy, the first year of analysis often witnesses unconscious efforts by the patient to manipulate the analyst into providing gratification and security according to long-standing fantasies of controlling the object of dependency. Such wishful fantasies of what can best be described as "magical control" may not be revealed openly in briefer nonanalytic psychotherapy and may not have the exaggerated intensity so often found in psychoanalysis. Psychotherapy is more controlled and circumscribed by the therapist than is psychoanalysis. In the latter, greater demands consequently fall upon the analyst for unwavering self-examination and self-understanding, for patience and for vigilance for signs that the patient is becoming excessively anxious owing to desires, impulses and emotions that shame and humiliate him or her. Helpless rage is also more likely to occur during analysis if the patient interprets as a rejection the abstinence and the frustration necessarily imposed by the analyst's effort to avoid gratifying infantile wishes.

This patient received the analyst assigned to her with a mixture of wariness and anticipation. The analyst, a relatively inexperienced man, approached her with naive enthusiasm but soon found himself somewhat overwhelmed by his patient's unexpected outpouring of erotic fantasies and by her unconscious seductiveness, which deflected her attention from what he considered the best purposes of the treatment. After a few weeks of being noncommittal, he "interpreted" her behavior during treatment as an attempt, in fantasy, to have the analyst replace three lost love objects—her fiance, her father, and the elder brother who had occasionally protected her.

As soon as she recognized her analyst's discomfort and withdrawal in response to her erotic fantasies, she began having dreams of repeated failure and inadequacy. The physical symptoms, which had begun to subside after a week of daily sessions, promptly flared up with alarming intensity. The tenor of her associations changed from pleasurable fantasies of marriage to the analyst to fears of certain rejection by every man because of her illness and its repellent symptoms. Hopelessness about her damaged femininity became the theme of her analytical sessions in the hospital. She felt that she was unattractive and that even the analyst was disgusted by her. Her depression grew more severe. Underlying the despairing complaints was an intensified hostility toward anyone in the hospital, whether staff member, nurse or patient, who failed to satisfy her demands for service, consideration and special regard. The patient watched closely for signs of criticism or displeasure in her analyst, but his renewed tolerance and unquestioning acceptance of her accusations during this opening phase of treatment gradually counteracted her anger at him and her excessive guilt.

For two weeks, however, her physical symptoms were as severe as they had ever been. The analyst tried to maintain an outward calm and optimism, but his personal anxiety and doubt about her analyzability increased. Fortunately, she seemed not to have detected his doubts; her disappointed rage at the futility of turning her wishful sexual fantasies into reality began to subside. Her diarrhea also remitted, and within another week she had definitely begun to improve. There continued to be brief interruptions in her increasingly lengthening remissions, which demonstrated the interaction between certain emotional conflicts and somatic reactions. For example, an older sister-in-law who had agreed to pay the patient's hospital expenses visited her and piously stated that she hoped the patient had "learned her lesson" and would henceforth curb her extravagance—implying also that she should not depend on her family so much. The patient suppressed her anger at the criticisms, which were not unjustified, and her diarrhea became severe. The analyst was able, however, to evoke an emotional verbal display of her feelings of rage during her session, and the somatic symptoms subsided in a few days.

A more dramatic episode occurred in the hospital ward. A patient in the next bed persisted in playing a radio loudly and in borrowing her belongings without permission. After some weeks of politely remonstrating the woman, the patient expressed her complaints in analysis. The sympathy of her analyst helped her to release her rage through an explosive outburst in the ward. She astonished her nurses by smashing the radio and screaming vituperations at her offending neighbor. Ordinarily, such violence would have induced her to experience remorse, shame and a prompt return of somatic symptoms. This time, her analyst's tacit support and noncritical attitude seemed to ward off most of the physical reaction. After a brief relapse, she made a rapid recovery and was discharged from the hospital in a few weeks. The remission was not quite complete, however, since she still had several semiformed stools a day, but no bleeding.

Improvement had begun with a subtle change in the patient's attitude toward the analyst. Her fantasy of a love affair became one of a close collaboration with him. Simultaneously, her thoughts turned to her past relationships. In reviewing the conflicts with her siblings and their wives, she bestowed less blame on them and experienced fewer feelings of martyrdom; she recalled how she would turn to her father for comfort and how she had feared displeasing or hurting him; and she vividly relived her power struggles with her unstable and domineering mother. It was evident to the analyst that she had tried to replace her father with him and had for a moment enacted secret fantasies of having her father all to herself. After the first premature one, no further effort was made for a long time to interpret her unconscious projection upon the analyst of the forbidden fantasies of childhood. Her hopes of becoming special and of gaining unique virtues through her relationship to the analyst were not destroyed. Many months were to elapse before more realistic insights would become tolerable to her. Fortunately, her *immediate* physical improvement did not depend upon her gaining insight. Inner calm and relief from the hopelessness about resolving her conflicts were temporarily achieved through dependence upon her analyst and through the unconscious fantasy that she might win his love in the future. The security created by this dependence was sufficient to relieve the overactivity of her colon and to block the psychological regression that had led her to express intense emotions by physical discharge instead of by thoughts and words.

The initial phase of her analysis was essentially a period of abreaction of her anger with the tacit encouragement of the analyst. In so doing, he laid the groundwork for a better working relationship between them. The patient slowly began to trust him more and to tolerate the kind of comments that her extreme sensitivity in the beginning of analysis had misinterpreted as censure and disapproval. The analyst, by his supportive interventions during the first phase, served as an auxiliary conscience ("superego") that was in time able to mitigate the harshness of her own self-critical judgments. These self-punitive attitudes reflected the reproduction of her mother's unreasonable and sadistic attacks upon her and of her own convictions about her essential "badness." The ideals she unconsciously set for herself were not realistic but represented fantasies of how to win parental love and devotion. Since they seemed unattainable, each new failure let loose a barrage of self-punishment that found expression in her destructive disease. The illness also offered an unassailable excuse for her regression to helpless dependence upon her family and others. As the incident with her sister-in-law showed, her pathetic state did not prevent her caretakers from displaying snide holier-than-thou attitudes, which provoked more helpless rage that remained unexpressed.

Interpretive comments by the analyst were limited to clarifying how the patient perpetuated feelings of helplessness and ultimately of hopelessness by responding to the aggressive demands of others with either silence or counteraggression. The analyst did not challenge her tendency to project her own hostile attitudes upon others. She would blame them for imaginary cruelty that in fact reflected her own savage impulses, of which she was totally unaware. The analyst inferred the existence of such impulses from her occasional slips of the tongue, her dreams and repeated aspects of behavior toward persons close to her. In "unplanned" ways she managed to frustrate or hurt them despite her insistent claims of having the best intentions.

After leaving the hospital, she resumed her therapy in the analyst's private office. She began to use the couch, giving up eye contact with her therapist and the distraction it provided from introspection and from free association of ideas.

As her strength returned, she spoke of actively engaging in a search for work, which the analyst supported. She still had periods of mild diarrhea. Despite the improvement, the patient was phobic about leaving the vicinity of the toilet, fearing a loss of sphincter control. Nevertheless, she recognized the need to become self-sufficient and financially independent.

The next months witnessed her struggle to overcome her child-like wish to remain helpless and passive. Her job-hunting met with one discouraging failure after another. When the analyst stated that he suspected that she arranged her own rejections, she complained indignantly that he was unfair and cruel to think anything of the sort. Angry outbursts at him were usually followed by self-denunciation for "being like mother." Each time the analyst mentioned her unconscious resistance to becoming independent, anger and a return of diarrhea followed. The analyst offered the interpretation that perhaps she was reexperiencing the fears of separation from her unresponsive parents that she had endured as a child when ill. He noted the similarity of her rage at his doubt that her need to remain helpless was genuine to her bitterness at the skepticism of her mother and brothers about her childhood ailments. She slowly recognized how skillfully she had discouraged prospective employers. She would insist on being "honest" by describing her recent illness to them in unnecessary detail! She "reassured" them that, while not fully recovered, she would "soon" regain all her strength. Six months after her hospitalization, she finally got a chance to work. At once a steady flow of complaints and expressions of martyrdom began. She stated, "No one helps me. My supervisor can't be satisfied; she expects too much. Nobody appreciates how much I do in spite of my illness. Of course you [the analyst] think I should go on, and I will have to put up with it all. I hope you're right." Each bout of helpless anger at the ordinary demands of her job, at criticism for slowness or inefficiency or at lack of recognition when she did well continued to be followed by a flare-up of bloody diarrhea. The analyst privately feared that he might indeed be expecting too much, but trusting in the strength of her positive attachment to him, he resolutely supported her efforts. Despite difficult times, she did not stop working.

Her fantasies and dreams gradually changed in content. Resentment, painful suffering and despair gave way to a repetition of the erotic fantasies and daydreams about her analyst with which she had begun her therapy in the hospital. With shame, she confessed to masturbating to thoughts of her analyst. He made no comment, and she apparently took his reaction to be noncritical. During the next three months, she had no more than three or four semiformed stools a day. Periodically, when angry at her family or her new employers, she would threaten to give up working. One crisis occurred when the brother and sister-in-law with whom she had lived after leaving the hospital found it necessary to move to another part of the country. For a time, she raged in despair at their "desertion." She stubbornly fought the analyst's efforts to relate her current need for parental caretakers to her early and futile struggle to compel her mother to provide unquestioning devotion. Each such interpretation was met by tears and by furious denials that her expectations were too high.

Nevertheless, the analyst's patient clarifications of her distortions of the real meaning of ongoing situations slowly lightened her depression and moderated her barely repressed rage. She found her own apartment and began to enjoy new-found freedom. She cultivated new friends and became less oppositional and less complaining at work. By the end of the first 16 months of therapy, the quality of her communications in the analysis as well as its content had begun to change. The first phase of her analytical therapy could be described as depressive-paranoid; the patient's primary interest was seeking and holding on to infant-like dependent ties to parent substitutes. She remained incapable of returning mature affection and fulfilling its responsibilities. People she loved were primarily instruments that provided safety and simple gratification.

The second phase of the analysis roughly paralleled the normal stage of psychological growth seen in the second, third and fourth years of life, when the child moves to separate itself from its mother's control and to practice mastery over its own actions. Peers become more important; rivalry and competition are now stronger motivating forces; genital sexual needs are more sharply focused; ideals and conscience grow stronger; and behavior is better controlled without the threats and intervention of external authorities. The second phase of the patient's analysis was also a phase of development of independence and a stronger individuality; it marked the beginning of her genuine separation from mothering figures. Her obsessive-compulsive ways of controlling anger at frustrations and her immature sexual aims and aggressive attitudes were revealed. The task of the analysis during this phase was to demonstrate these aspects of character to the patient convincingly enough to motivate her to alter them.

For a time in the second phase, her associations became paradoxically less spontaneous and less emotionally expressive but more wordy and circumstantial. She admitted that it had suddenly become more difficult to speak freely to her analyst. Whereas the first phase of analysis was dominated by her regression to child-like dependency and by her projection of hostile feelings upon others, which permitted her to disown her own aggression, the second phase was marked by intellectualization, isolation of feelings that became difficult to identify and conversion of those feelings that did emerge into their opposites: Hate became protective concern, frustration and rage became disappointment and hurt, pleasure-seeking was replaced by duty and obligation, and passivity was converted into stubborn efforts to control others.

Fortunately for the analysis, her dreams, which had become richer in content and more frequent, provided a transparent gateway to understanding the true desires and feelings behind her "reaction formations." The analysis of her dreams over the next two years gradually gave her an undeniable understanding of how she turned attitudes and emotions into their opposites. For example, she warded off a return of the extreme dependence and helplessness that had accompanied her severe attack of ulcerative colitis by adopting an exaggerated independence. She reacted to her conviction of having been cheated of maternal love by assuming fanatical dedication to tolerance and justice for everyone. She reversed her infantile symbiotic tendencies by going out of her way to adopt "lame ducks," by which she meant men who were "losers" or otherwise disabled.

The model for this more independent self-image and its changed ideals and aims proved to be an identification with her father. By identifying with him as a self-sacrificing leader, she diminished the need for dependent attachments to a powerful mother surrogate, and, at the same time, intensified the attachment to her analyst. He and her father were equated, and the wish to be like them strengthened her against the pathogenic emotional states caused by her futile attachments to women, whom she managed invariably to antagonize and to alienate. For a long time, the balance between tendencies toward masculine identification and those toward helpless dependence remained precarious. Frequent relapses to the old state of dependence occurred whenever she believed that she would be deserted by or separated from the most important person of the moment.

Identification with paternal qualities of self-sufficiency and devotion to others also countered her guilt for being a "bad girl" and muted the resultant self-destructive impulses. During analysis, she broadened the base of her identification to include other desirable qualities, such as patience, tolerance and recognition of her limitations. These were associated with "real" qualities of the analyst that she had repeatedly experienced directly and in time came to idealize.

This new state of the analysis was marked by steady reduction of bowel symptoms and by objective evidence of remission of the inflammatory process in the colon. The change confirmed the analyst's initial impression—that somatic "expression" by the colon of her conflicts and the emotions induced by them was directly related to helplessness and hopelessness about coping with serious frustration or loss. That state of helpless despair in turn aroused a latent need for a more complete symbiotic-like dependence upon an omnipotent mothering person.

The second phase of the analysis was "announced" with a dream: "I seemed to be seeing or visiting my father, who was apparently away in another city, working. I waited in his house for him. The people there said he was so popular. The men remarked, 'That was some blonde he ran around with.' It seemed that mother had been dead a long time. I felt we were all grown up and that he was living his own life."

Her thoughts revolved around her affection for and sexual fantasies about the analyst, jealousy of his private life and feelings of being unattractive to him. (The blonde in her dream was a woman analyst she had seen conversing with the analyst a few days earlier.) She "guessed" that her feelings about him must be connected with her father. Perhaps, she mused, being alone led her to turn to the analyst for love, as she had once tried to do with her father. Recognizing that the patient's view of herself and her relations with others might be changing, the analyst chose not to introduce at this time any distracting and disturbing references to repressed and still frightening incestuous fantasies.

A remission began, during which the patient reviewed the positive aspects of her ties to her father and the evidence that he had indeed loved her. After two weeks of no diarrhea, she reported another dream: "Dr. X came to me for help; he looked very tired. He seemed ill and asked me to take his temperature, but his thermometers were peculiar. One was twice as long as a pencil and thicker; the other was a small solid medicine dropper with the curved tip broken off. I couldn't read the big one, and the other was worthless. He said he had a call to make and would return. I felt baffled and sorry because it seemed such a simple thing to do. His child came in and said to hurry up, was I going to take all night."

She identified Dr. X as a hospital physician of whom she had been fond. Her associations led to her convictions that everyone had always expected the impossible from her and had exploited her and that men tried to assign her the masculine role of looking after them. Her fiance had been such a passive but demanding man. The analyst wondered whether she might not have *chosen* her men for that very reason; perhaps she preferred men to be weak and dependent upon her. With this intervention, the analyst was attempting to bring forward fantasies that she had repressed out of shame and in fear of a dreaded retaliation by men for wishing to take their place. The patient became indignant and said angrily that the analyst was accusing her cruelly and unfairly of *wanting to be a man*. She became moderately depressed, and her diarrhea returned.

Despite her vehement denials, counterattacks and recurring diarrhea, she nevertheless continued to think of the analyst's comment and to associate it with forgotten incidents that indicated that he had been correct. For several weeks, she struggled with this new but unwelcome image of herself. Her dreams revealed more of her unconscious wish to be a man and to have a penis. She felt a helpless resentment at having been born a girl; she envied men and their special privileges. She saw her sex as the reason for her mother's contempt and rejection. Her depression deepened. She began to speak of fears of death and in dreams represented herself as a dying child abandoned by its mother.

The depression and the diarrhea continued several weeks. She was encouraged to continue working despite her symptoms. A new trend finally began with the following dream: "The dream had two parts. First, I was sliding up and down a totem pole. Next, I was walking through the woods with my brothers. I stopped to look at a bright red fungus growth on the trunk of a tree. I had a strong impulse to tear it off and keep it. But I didn't and hurried back to my brothers."

She immediately recalled the dream of Dr. X in which she had been required to play the masculine role of the doctor without usable equipment. She then thought of her chronic unhappiness at not receiving praise and of her efforts to compete with fellow workers in her present job, which reminded her of her long and bitter quarrels with her brothers. Did this last dream, she wondered, mean that she had wanted to hurt them, perhaps to kill them? After all, to castrate them (to tear off the growth on the tree) would be like killing them.

Her analyst agreed with her interpretation of her aggressive castrative impulses. She stated that she felt that the totem pole sequence expressed her wish to have her father and his penis all for herself. The idea of such intense violent competition for her father, not only with her siblings but also with her mother, horrified her. Guilt and depression deepened, and her diarrhea grew worse. The analyst stated that her diarrhea signified her futile aggressive feelings toward rivals. Loss of the power to control events and persons close to her led to the general sense of helplessness and depression that fostered her regression once again to a symbiotic-like dependence. Here the vicious circle became complete. No one could tolerate her helpless attachments without becoming critical and withdrawing. The futile anger and guilt intensified, and the diarrhea took over as her primary nonverbal mode of expressing negative feelings about herself as well as about the "mothers" who continually rejected her.

Despite her depression and the exacerbation of colitis, the patient struggled to keep working and, to her analyst's surprise, even improved her work effectiveness. She began to receive praise, was promoted and was given a raise. These unexpected rewards reinforced the analyst's interpretations of the impact upon her health of emotional factors. Within two weeks she began to have dreams of eating and of being fed, and for the first time in more than a month, the colitis improved. Fantasies of an infant-like attachment to a mothering woman were replaced by the wish for a strong, loving man like her father or her analyst whom she could help in his work. This trend roughly marked the end of the transitional second phase of the analysis.

The third phase lasted until the termination of analytical therapy three years later. It was marked by a freer and more expressive use of words rather than colon activity to convey emotional reactions. The analytical process now assumed a course and a content typical of the usual psychoanalytical treatment of a psychoneurosis.

The patient interpreted the depressions, now relatively mild and short-lived, as a retreat from competitive struggles to what she ruefully called "back to mother." In a serious effort to identify deep-seated sexual conflicts that had begun in early childhood, she recalled how her mother had publicly shamed her when she caught her masturbating ("rubbing herself"). To gain acceptance by her mother, she had "arranged" to lose out with boys and men as the expiation for her "bad" sexual impulses. She described her dilemma in the following dream:

"I was with young people walking, at a school or club. I came to an escalator leading down to a pool. I felt I wanted to learn to swim; I should have long ago. I was terribly afraid of the escalator but forced myself down. Someone asked why I looked so strange. A boy laughed at me and asked what did I have against escalators. A boy I admired was going to teach me to swim. I wanted to go back and put on my swimming clothes. I began running, but everything kept interrupting. An old crippled lady wanted me to walk with her; the director of the club gave me a job to do. I finally got back, panicky that the boy would be gone. I recalled I had always feared the water, but not with this boy. He was waiting but was angry. I tried to explain, but he did not believe my story and he left me."

Her recollections went back to early sex play at age four or five with a neighbor's young son. She had been discovered by one of her brothers, who had promptly reported her to their mother. Reliving the unforgiving fury of her mother, she suddenly wondered if her analyst was not equally disgusted by her.

On the next night she dreamed: "I was having to submit to the loss of an eye for my mother. The doctor said she was going blind and that the only thing was to remove one of my eyes and give it to her. Everybody in the family agreed it should be done. I felt it was unfair, but since they all agreed I couldn't object."

The first dream, she said, referred to her fears of sex and to her sexual frustration, which she blamed on her family's demands. In the second, she felt that her "castration," in the form of an "eye for an eye," represented an obligation to her mother. She recalled how often her mother had blamed her daughter's birth during her early menopause for the disabling illnesses that plagued her and interfered with her own sexual life. Now, sexual needs drove the patient to deny herself gratification, as she had "denied" it to her mother.

For the next few weeks, she had anxiety dreams of being bombed and attacked in other ways. Finally, she reported a waking experience that associated sexual excitement and the anxiety it caused her with increased bowel activity. She recalled that a day before the two dreams just mentioned, she had suffered a brief period of abdominal pain that seemed to radiate from her genitals. "I had been in bed and had felt sexual tension but had not masturbated. I feel asleep and dreamed of being shot at. When I awoke I felt less sexual arousal but for the next day had much gas and a constant desire to move my bowels; there was no stool, only a little mucus." Her associations were concerned with fellatio and a desire to be "filled up by a man's penis." On the other hand, it meant getting a man's "masculinity—not just pleasure, but his power, his worth and his pride in himself."

Months of repetitive working on this aggressive oral sexual theme followed. Periodically, the slow rate of change produced complaints of futility mixed with outbursts of resentment at the analyst for expecting too much of her. The colitis, however, was not reactivated. When the question of ending analysis was broached by the patient and agreed to by the analyst after more than five years of treatment, there was a minor flare-up of constipation and diarrhea. She admitted that the prospect of termination frightened her. Losing the analyst and perhaps never marrying depressed her, but she was no longer helpless or hopeless about her life. The analysis ended at a set date.

SUMMARY

The patient was followed almost 20 years. She remained free of ulcerative colitis symptoms, and repeated bowel studies revealed no evidence of disease. She suffered from occasional headaches and backaches; she did not marry but occasionally became infatuated with men who were either unhappily married or physically ill. She continued to work and support herself. Difficulties with women in authority still occurred. She was unhappy at times but no longer suffered severe depression.

The effects of the analysis were mixed. Her basic masochistic character was not materially changed, although the intensity of her need for suffering was certainly diminished. The analysis had not fully succeeded in improving her enjoyment of sex and undoing her long-standing inhibition. She seldom seemed genuinely happy and trusting in a sexual relationship with a strong and self-sufficient man. Consequently, her sexual relationships continued to be structured in terms of dominance and submission; she now generally played the controlling role. The analysis had substantially strengthened her identifications with her father as a self-sacrificing leader and with the idealized image of the analyst as a giving person. Most significantly for her physical health, her tendency to regress and to become excessively dependent had clearly been halted. Presumably, the stronger masculine identification and her firmer ideal image of herself as independent warded off the dangerous regression to a helpless attachment to a mothering figure. That in turn reduced the danger of an emotional regression to the "language of the colon," which one might call the "mother" tongue of symbiosis in cases such as this.

Case Two: Psychotherapy by Support and Catharsis with Prolonged Medical-Psychiatric Follow-up

The patient was a woman first seen at the Presbyterian Hospital (New York) when she was 26 years old. Emotional factors in her ulcerative colitis were clear-cut. Intermittent psychotherapy over an eight-year period was productive, and her change of environment led to a dramatic remission. The case is especially significant because of the medical-psychiatric follow-up of 47 years.

The patient was first seen in consultation during her first admission, which was, however, during her fourth attack. The first attack had occurred in 1924, nine months after she had started a business venture that caused her worry and financial strain. She recovered from a relatively mild attack of bloody diarrhea after spending a month at a local spa on the advice of her physician.

She showed the dependence on family members characteristic of patients with ulcerative colitis. She was the seventh and youngest child of a Southern black family. Her mother died when she was two-and-a-half years old, and she was subsequently sent to live with an aunt who treated her badly. At eight years of age she was sent North to live with a married sister, whom she later helped support.

A traumatic sexual experience occurred that involved this sister. Shortly after the patient reached puberty, her brother-in-law seduced her and threatened to kill her if she told his wife. She became pregnant, however, and confided in her sister. An abortion was performed, and her sister left her husband. The patient continued to brood and to feel guilty about her role in the break-up for many years; she also feared that she had contracted syphilis. While still young she had two opportunities to marry, but in each instance she broke off the relationship for fear that her earlier sexual experience would be discovered.

The attack that first brought her to the hospital psychiatrist was provoked by a conflict that was to remain an important factor in the eight years of psychiatric observation and treatment.

She was then living with another older sister who was divorced and had a 10-year-old child. The patient was in business with this sister and shared expenses. She resented the sister for not compelling her former husband to support them, which forced the patient to assume much of the responsibility for them as well as for other family members. She was fond of music, but the added family burdens prevented her from progressing in her musical training. Prior to the attack requiring hospitalization, she had been negotiating with her current employer for a transfer to the company's branch in the far West, primarily to escape from the family situation. She had even bought her tickets when she again became ill. She remarked, "I suppose the excitement was too much."

The patient had three hospitalizations during the following year. These attacks were characterized by severe bloody diarrhea, vomiting, weight loss, arthritic symptoms and spiking temperatures. Proctoscopic examination showed a marked hyperemia of the mucous membrane, with shallow ulcers of various sizes. Secondary anemia was severe and required several transfusions.

The patient was seen by the psychiatrist five times during the three hospitalizations, most often after the first admission. At the initial consultation, the immediate conflict with her sister and her background as an orphan were explored. The second visit came five days later at the patient's request, during which she confessed to the sexual encounter with her brother-in-law and to the abortion. Most of the other interviews were brief and dealt with the situation with her sister, who interfered with her practicing the piano, criticized her friends and discouraged their coming to the apartment. The therapist listened sympathetically as she complained about her sister. She decided to stay in New York for at least another year. The patient stated that the absence of men in her life did not bother her; what she could not tolerate was "to be angry." The ventilation of her rage became one of the chief aims of subsequent therapeutic sessions, in addition to allaying her sense of guilt.

Two years after her first admission, she became an out-patient at the psychotherapist's request. She related an incident of a year before, in which a burglar had entered the apartment and stolen her sister's pocketbook. The patient again became anxious, and her diarrhea returned; she remained in bed three months, attended by her internist and her sister.

During the out-patient interview, she reported that she was back at work, was going to occasional concerts and was interested in art and philanthropic organizations. She occasionally dated a male friend but considered it a waste of time that could have been devoted to cultural interests. She continued to complain about her sister, who was inclined to disparage everything she was trying to do. She questioned whether she should leave her sister and the sister's child, whom she was now largely supporting. She was gently encouraged by the therapist to move away from her sister.

After five months, she looked well and reported that she was symptom-free. She had been working since the previous October and was reconciled to staying in New York and assisting her sister, but she had not entirely given up the idea of going to the West Coast. She was not being seen regularly at this time and did not keep a follow-up appointment six weeks later.

The following year, she was again admitted to the hospital because of severe backache, anorexia and general malaise. Her arthritic symptoms had returned, and just before admission bloody diarrhea reappeared.

Psychiatric consultation was again requested. Because the situation at home had become unbearable, she had sought an apartment of her own. She had just found one that suited her when her symptoms recurred.

It seemed imperative to begin more intensive psychotherapy, and it was recommended that she come regularly once a week for six weeks. A medical follow-up showed her "bowels behaving." She did not keep her psychiatric appointments, and the therapist received a long letter from her explaining why: She had had a return of arthritic symptoms, had been in bed part of the time, had had two teeth pulled, and so forth. She stated that she would phone for an appointment when she felt better.

One of the striking features of this patient's psychotherapy was its irregularity. Whenever an attempt was made to deal with separation from her sister, she interrupted treatment. When the therapist saw her again about two years later, she said that a year before she had decided not to go to any doctors and had tried Christian Science instead, with some success! She had been working steadily, but because another crisis with her sister had developed, she had rented a small one-and-a-half room apartment, into which she planned to move in a few months. She was given every encouragement to go ahead with her plan to separate and was given an appointment for the next week. She broke the appointment and wrote that her plans to move into the new apartment "went haywire." The management had demanded advance rent, which she felt unable to pay. She finished her letter by stating that she might leave New York. In another letter, several months later, she wrote that she had finally taken the step that she had been trying to make for years: She at least had her own apartment. There had been many unpleasant scenes with her sister, but she had held her own, despite experiencing some depression. Nine months later, she was seen in the out-patient clinic because, following her move away from her sister, she had suffered from dizziness. The sister had been unpleasant and had harassed her during her efforts to become independent. She had had no recurrence of her diarrhea as in the past. Six months later, she reported that she had finally triumphed in the battle with her sister: The patient moved her piano to her own apartment. She felt that she "would go crazy" and had spells of dizziness and gastric disturbances. There was no diarrhea, however. The final crisis had come when her sister had attempted to compel her to return the piano. Suddenly the patient found herself swearing at her sister and "standing up for her rights." The sister continued to berate her, even bringing up the matter of the patient's unfortunate sexual experience as a child. With this, the patient "hit the ceiling" and excoriated the sister violently for this unfair attack. Although shaken by the experience, the patient felt much relieved.

The following year, the therapist received word from her that she had finally moved to a Western city, was improved and had gained weight. This was followed by a detailed letter in which she discussed her problems in adjusting to the new environment, and in which she enclosed a clipping from a local New York newspaper reviewing her career with the firm for which she had worked 10 years. It included a remark her employer had made to her on her leaving: "I've opened the doors of the West for you—now it's up to you." This was to be a time of real advancement in her career, without further interference from the colitis.

A brief comment about the psychotherapy carried out sporadically over the eight-year period in New York may be made. During that time, she was seen by the therapist on only 14 occasions, both during her hospitalizations and as an out-patient. There were periods of a year at a time when she avoided the therapist. Nevertheless, she always felt that the therapist remained interested in her. One telling connection was her periodic exchange of letters with him. During their personal contacts, she was encouraged to express her resentment and hostility toward her sister and received full support from the therapist regarding the justice of her cause. She was also encouraged to establish herself independently. Her resistance to intensive therapy was recognized, and she was not pressured in any way. Her core conflict, needs for dependency versus guilt, was repeatedly and dramatically illustrated by her repeated behaviors. Clearly there was dependence on a mother substitute—her older sister—accentuated by her early orphaning. She was obliged to work through this before she could leave New York and, in so doing, put an end to her attacks of ulcerative colitis.

A follow-up note is of interest. Six years after leaving her sister, while on a visit to New York, she was interviewed by the therapist. She described her initial loneliness on first moving to the West Coast and the racial prejudice against which she was compelled to struggle most painfully. Matters gradually improved, and she became a considerable success in her profession. At the time she was seen, she had set up her own shop, which she proudly said was patronized by important figures. She was active in promoting better racial understanding, was voted the person who had contributed most to the war effort in her community and was even given a medal. Medical examination at this time showed no disease in the colon.

The patient was then lost to follow-up for the next 12 years. Quite by accident, the therapist discovered her on a television program, in connection with an exhibit of her work.

The therapist wrote to the patient, and she replied with a long letter that described her life since 1946. Her shop, a great success, had continued to be patronized by the elite. She closed this successful business after the deaths of her sister in New York and of her brother. Though depressed for a period, she seemed not to have experienced a return of diarrhea. After closing the shop, she had been sought for other prestigious positions, which she had taken.

She still found some difficulty in expressing anger but on several occasions had done so effectively.

The patient reported that she had had no bowel disturbances in these preceding five years.

With the exceptions of her family problems and her unmarried status, the changes in her life had been fortuitous and clearly for the better. It should not be overlooked that they were mainly changes she had brought about herself. The patient felt that psychiatric treatment had helped her greatly and that she had learned to study herself and to be more patient with others. She was not preoccupied with her illness, was able to relax more than before, and felt that she was more active socially and better able to express her anger, although not without experiencing some guilt.

Her greatest inhibitions seemed to be in the sexual area, about which she withheld detailed information. She had recently had an opportunity to marry but was unable to do so—she had convinced herself that to marry would be the worst thing she could "have done for myself and to myself." The final psychiatric diagnosis was obsessive personality disorder with reactive depressive trends. By this time, the patient had been free of her ulcerative colitis 24 years.

In 1971, it was learned that in 1963 she had undergone a partial colectomy for carcinoma of the colon. Four years later, she was found to have a rectal carcinoma that required an abdominoperineal resection with partial resection of the vagina; an ileostomy was established in the right lower quadrant. The ileal stoma functioned well, and she said it was not a serious problem.

In 1972, she wrote that she was now retired and remained close to her home, enjoying T.V. and her collection of records. She made the statement, "All in all God has been good to me, in spite of everything and I am most grateful. Have been interested in Science for many years and am truly grateful for the mental help and peace of mind it has given to me." She ended by expressing her gratitude for the contribution that the Columbia-Presbyterian Medical Center had made and especially for the therapist's unflagging interest in her.

The dynamic forces that altered the patient's emotional life are fairly transparent in this case. She suffered from an intense need for maternal love and protection, while simultaneously being threatened by an equally intense fear of rejection and even of exploitation by those on whom she sought to depend. Her repressed rage at failing to be appreciated, despite her shows of self-sacrifice, induced an ever-present sense of guilt that could only be made endurable by arranging pain and suffering, a form of self-punishment. The colitis represented both a substitute for the unexpressed rage at her sister and the suffering she needed and seemed to feel she deserved. In fact, suffering through illness was her only way of extracting concern from her sister. It goes without saying that her early sexual "transgression" merely increased her sense of guilt.

The therapist represented the magical, powerful, healing medical institution that "mothered her" without asking anything in return; but at a more personal level, he became an auxiliary conscience that helped her defy her own conscience, which seemed always ready to echo her sister's accusations against her.

Thus, although the therapist's contacts may have been tenuous, through letters and telephone conversations he was able to maintain a steady support that remained at least a partial source of strength for more than 40 years.

Case Three: Psychotherapy of a Case of Ulcerative Colitis Associated With Hysterical Depression

This case has been selected because of certain dramatic features in the history and because of the clear interrelationship between psychical factors and physical reactions. It is illustrative also of a coordinated medical, surgical, psychiatric and social treatment program for a severe case of ulcerative colitis, carried out for nearly five years.

The patient was a 32-year-old housewife who had had three attacks of ulcerative colitis and was first seen by a psychiatrist during her fourth recurrence. The patient's first episode occurred at the age of 18 years and coincided with problems in her courtship; it cleared up after she had spent six weeks in a hospital. The second attack occurred after initial signs of fatal heart disease appeared in her favorite brother. This attack, too, was of short duration but was followed by a more severe one four months later. In the meantime, she had married, and her brother had died. This third attack occurred on the anniversary of her brother's birthday, when a monument was erected at his grave.

The patient had two pregnancies between the third attack and the fourth attack of ulcerative colitis. The first pregnancy was associated with unusual circumstances. She displayed a lack of interest both in this and in her second pregnancy; in neither case did she make any preparations for the child. She claimed that she had not felt the quickening of the first child until the seventh month, and then only if she made a definite effort. She later became aware that she had frequently risked having a miscarriage owing to her "habit" of bearing down on urinating in the later months of pregnancy.

In the ninth month of the first pregnancy, she complained tearfully to her husband that she could not urinate but denied that this could be a sign of labor. When her difficulty occurred a second time, her husband ignored her protests and called an ambulance. During the next few minutes, the patient, in attempting to urinate, expelled her live infant into the toilet bowl. A physician arrived in time to deliver the placenta. There were accusations made that she and her husband had deliberately drowned the baby. The physician could not believe the truth—that a profoundly hysterical patient had no realization that her straining had delivered an infant. The whole episode had taken barely 15 minutes and, aside from a few moments of palpitation, she had experienced no marked discomfort. As is typical of hysteria, amnesia by repression created the bizarre tragedy. Later in psychotherapy, she was to recall details that she had repressed.

For the next few months, the patient was depressed and avoided meeting any of her friends, to whom she had earlier announced her anticipation of the coming child. She continually saw the vision of the dead baby being held up by the doctor, and she went over again and again the remarks made by the physicians. Eager to have another child, she consulted a doctor, who told her that she could become pregnant but should wait six months, which she did. During this pregnancy, her depression was no longer consciously present.

In the second pregnancy, she developed tachycardia with her first labor pains. After she arrived at the hospital, labor was induced owing to the continued tachycardia, and she was delivered of a living male child. She had complete amnesia for 12 hours preceding delivery and partial amnesia for two days following, about which she remarked, "It seemed a question of fifteen minutes and not at all two days." Both the anesthetic miscarriage and this amnesia appear to have been hysterical. Her delivery did not stop the tachycardia, and because cardiac collapse was feared, a cardiologist was called in. The family reported that the patient did not seem at all aware of the seriousness of her condition: She asked how the baby was and remarked what an easy labor she had had. The patient later compared her speech and manner with those of her brother just before his death. During the last few days in the hospital, she felt well, and she was discharged in 10 days to her mother's home.

Three days after she returned home from the hospital, bloody diarrhea marked the start of the fourth attack of ulcerative colitis. Three weeks later, a series of continuing arguments with her mother, who also seemed prone to exaggerate the patient's slightest ailments, ended in an episode in which the patient fainted upon urinating and had paroxysmal tachycardia that necessitated her return to the hospital.

Three months after the beginning of this attack, she was admitted to the Presbyterian Hospital, where she remained for five months. She averaged daily 12 stools containing blood and pus. A barium enema 10 days after admission showed an absence of the usual haustral markings in the transverse, descending and ascending colons. The evidence of marked colonic disorder was consistent with the clinical diagnosis of chronic ulcerative colitis.

Ten days after admission, she had another attack of paroxysmal tachycardia associated with precordial pain. It is noted in the chart that the patient was crying and tremendously apprehensive, "having, unfortunately, been told on the outside that unless an attack could be controlled 'within 48 hours' it would be fatal." This attack was controlled by vagal pressure. Ten days later, she had a second attack of tachycardia, again in unusual circumstances. The attack began while she was on the bedpan, and nothing that was tried, including drugs, could stop it. The patient's apprehension mounted as she reached the "deadline" of 48 hours. She watched the clock much of the time. Between the forty-seventh hour and the forty-eighth hour, the tachycardia subsided, and her pulse, which had reached as high as 205, again became regular. As the tachycardia subsided, it was replaced by pain beneath the sternum for which no explanation could be found.

It was after this series of unexplainable events that a psychiatric consultation was requested, a month and a half after her admission to the hospital. She was encouraged by her therapist to discharge affects freely during and between interviews, and her chest pain began to subside after several days and soon disappeared. As is characteristic of hysterical conversion symptoms, however, relief in one part of the body is often followed by a disorder appearing in another. In this case, her concern shifted to the anal area. She began to complain in the same way of the fistulae from which she had suffered for years. The hysterical reinforcement of the natural discomfort from the fistulae might have been successfully camouflaged if the shift had not been observed during psychotherapy. Such a psychical reinforcement of a naturally painful lesion is often difficult for the general practitioner or surgeon to interpret. It is usually argued that the patient has a perfect right to be upset, and the opportunity to evaluate and treat an important psychiatric complication is lost.

With further emotional catharsis, the more obvious sources of her complaints became evident. One was her disappointment that she was not at home to look after her second baby, who was now five months old. This was expressed in exaggerated form, an evident reaction formation to her rejection of the child; returning to it seemed more likely to intensify the diarrhea than to relieve it. She was gradually made to realize her mixed attitude toward the living child as the details of the first infant's death began to be made conscious.

Her resentment toward her husband was also quite consciously expressed and was directed chiefly at his inability to earn as a taxi driver what she considered an adequate income. She felt that life was hardly worthwhile without more comforts than they could afford. As treatment progressed, a more fundamental reason for her dislike of her husband became evident. Although willing, industrious and good-hearted, he was apparently of borderline intelligence and was illiterate and stupid in her eyes. She had sensed his inadequacies before marriage, but paradoxically they were the unconscious reasons for choosing him: He was a person whom she could care for and dominate intellectually. Nevertheless, she resented him because she could not depend upon him emotionally or get material comforts from him. He, however, loved her and the baby and exhibited many of the qualities of a large and faithful dog.

During her hospital residence, she repeatedly demonstrated the interrelationship between her emotional conflicts and her physical symptoms. Her husband's failure to bring in the usual sum of tips, a remark casually dropped by her father that she was getting well enough to be discharged soon, and the failure of her mother to visit her on a day when she had made an annual visit to the brother's grave each produced an acute exacerbation of symptoms.

Although the patient had little realization of it at this time, it soon became evident that the mother was in fact her most fundamental problem. Therefore, the necessity of the patient's eventually establishing her own home and for her to become active again was stressed to members of her family while she was still in the hospital. It was a year before the patient was ready for this step. At the end of six months, the patient was discharged to a convalescent home for a few weeks, after which she returned much improved to her parents' home.

She was now more antagonistic toward her husband; showed little interest in her baby, whom she feared she would injure; and frequently saw images of her dead brother, with whom she would carry on imaginary conversations. Because of her precarious mental and physical states and the strong probability that she might again have to be hospitalized unless matters changed, the therapist attempted a more intense method of psychotherapy. Periods of modified free association two or three times a week were inaugurated and were continued three-and-a-half months. This was not an attempt to conduct a psychoanalysis. The therapist attempted to keep from going too deeply. Association was directed instead of completely free. Recounting of dreams was not encouraged, and interpretations were made of only the more obvious situational factors, not of symbolic material that reflected primitive forbidden impulses.

The patient promptly began to develop choking sensations, with palpitation and anxiety. It had been explained to her while she was still in the hospital that it was likely as treatment progressed that palpitation would recur. This was a maneuver to anticipate the return of anxiety, which had preceded the more obvious conversion symptoms and which seemed likely to return before being resolved through catharsis and support. With the reappearance of anxiety, her diarrhea began to subside.

The most striking development during the first phase of "free" association was her discovery of her hostility toward her mother, of which she had been unaware, and which had served as one of the chief bonds of servitude and dependence. Her mother was a cantankerous woman who had become much more embittered following the death of her son. This son and the patient had always sided with the mother against other members of the family. The patient continued this attitude, upholding her mother against her father, and later either sided with her against her own husband or was torn by a conflict of loyalties. To illustrate the degree to which this went, she paraphrased the slogan, "My country, right or wrong," into "My mother, right or wrong." Recognizing that another person had justification for attacking her mother merely made her more vociferous in her defense of her mother. The deprivation that loss of love meant and its importance as a cause of physical disorders were illustrated in her relationship not only to her mother but also to mother surrogates.

During this three-and-a-half month period of free association, transference reactions became unmistakably evident. Her identification of the analyst with her dead brother came out in many ways. On the way to interviews, for example, she would imagine that it was her brother who was guiding her and who would see that she had the proper medicine and care. In time, through the transference, she was able to some degree to shift her attachment from a dead subject to a living one. The patient had one dream in which she came to see the psychiatrist with her husband, leading a nine-year-old boy whom she identified as her dead brother. The dream and subsequent associations disclosed historical material associated both with her brother (related to his soiling his pants) and with her husband (related to a quarrel and a reconciliation that had taken place). This and other evidence pointed to the conclusion that unconscious hostility toward this adored sibling also played an important role in her illness. It was not thought wise, however, to confront her with her dual feelings toward the beloved brother. Following this dream, her relationship to her husband much improved, and her positive attitude toward and love for him reasserted itself. This was the only dream spontaneously reported; as mentioned, relating dreams was not encouraged.

As her insight into her hostility toward significant persons increased, her negative attitude toward her mother was partly displaced to the surgical department and personnel of the hospital. She began to stand up for her and her husband's rights in the face of the family's, particularly the mother's, exploitation of her dependence and earlier submissiveness. It was clear that she had finally recognized the struggle that her mother would make to hold on to her when she stated that her mother would rather have her sick and at home than well and away. Such an attitude has proved to be not uncommon in the families of ulcerative colitis patients. Her family was furious with her, as might be expected, and they counted on her helplessness and on her past difficulty in supporting herself and the child to force her back into submission. During the quarrels that followed, she recalled with some apprehension that the diarrhea had begun a year before, after a protracted argument with her mother. She did not yield to her family, however, and for the first time she realized that she was able to live alone with her husband and baby in spite of her symptoms. After a few weeks of self-sufficiency, though, against her "better judgment" she did join the rest of the family at the beach because of the importuning of a brother that the others would not understand if she remained at home alone. She soon found the situation intolerable, but instead of submitting and falling ill, she accepted the challenge and gained added independence by openly expressing her resentment of the family's controlling attitude.

It is of interest that during that summer she had her first attack of hay fever and asthma. She was later found to be sensitive to ragweed and was treated for it. The allergic disturbance did not become prominent, but the appearance of asthma occurred at the time of separation from her mother. The triad of ulcerative colitis, disturbance of heart rhythm, and asthma has been encountered in other cases of ulcerative colitis, with one somatic syndrome often replacing another.

It now became possible to plan with her the best way to reestablish her own home. The patient's dependence on her mother had made it impossible to consider it practically earlier in treatment. It was necessary for the husband's earnings to be temporarily subsidized. Throughout the work with this patient, the Social Service Department had rendered invaluable service and was often symbolically a "good mother." Now this department provided financial help as a temporary aid over a three-and-a-half-year period. It was stopped when the husband obtained a job and salary commensurate with the economic needs of the family as an independent unit. It is doubtful whether the patient could have attained her later improvement if she had not been able to leave her mother's home and interfering control.

After moving in to her new home, the patient did not see the therapist for five months. Although not entirely symptom-free, she had learned to handle most disturbances herself. She had observed that emotional difficulties were most likely to bring a renewed frequency of stools. Provocative situations were now more likely to be directly confronted than repressed; the likelihood of prolonged recurrences was demonstrably lessened. Previous to psychotherapy, she had been unable to face her reactions to her husband's limitations. She had now also accepted that her child might not be as bright as some children. There were still conflicts about both issues, and her compulsive ideas about harming her child had not entirely disappeared. Nevertheless, they were at least more openly acknowledged, which made them less "toxic" psychologically.

Among the contraindications for surgery—and another argument for continuing conservative treatment as long as possible—is the nature of the patient's depressive mental trend. The colitis in this case, as in some other cases studied, appears to represent the expression of an unconscious suicidal trend, which is a powerful force working against recovery, and is easily set off by any adverse circumstances. We would expect, therefore, that convalescence from major surgery would be prolonged.

The nature of her unconscious thoughts and feelings was indicated by her reaction to a discussion with a surgeon about the possible necessity of surgery. Afterward she had a fantasy that in the following month, on the first anniversary of her father's death, her gravestone would appear next to his, and her friends would remark that hers was indeed an unfortunate family. This seemed to her to be the picture of an accomplished fact, which she contemplated without any particular affect. It was evident that the depression and her readiness for death were still active and potentially destructive despite the improvements made in her family and social adjustments.

The foregoing account covers 15 years of observations and periodic psychotherapy. The patient was followed regularly another 10 years and sporadically thereafter.

Six years after assuming her independence from her mother, the patient was admitted to the hospital for diarrhea and abdominal pain of three weeks' duration. The patient reported that she had been better the two previous years than at any time during her period of suffering from colitis.

When discharged, she was having five to eight bloody stools a day but was not losing weight. X-ray examination indicated involvement of the entire colon, with polyps in the descending colon and sigmoid. Owing to the patient's negative attitude toward radical surgery, a colectomy was postponed. By the next fall, however, the colitis had become more disabling, with abdominal pain as well as diarrhea, and she developed a rectovaginal fistula. A colectomy was advised and performed. The affected colon and the terminal portion of the ileum were excised, and an ileoanal anastomosis was done.

During the next year and a half, she continued to have frequent watery stools and severe abdominal pains, with some vomiting. The patient finally agreed to a permanent ileostomy, and the anal orifice was closed. This final piece of surgery occurred 26 years after the onset of her ulcerative colitis.

She expressed her gratitude toward the psychiatrist, who had helped her understand some of her problems, and who in particular had given her an awareness and appreciation of positive values in her life that had made living more tolerable.

Fortunately, the patient's adjustment to the ileostomy proved positive with the help and renewed encouragement of her first psychotherapist. She seemed more hopeful and began to take the initiative in caring for herself.

A year later, the patient presented a picture of health and contentment. That summer, for the first time since her marriage, she, her husband and her son spent a two-week vacation at the beach. Business was going well for her husband; they were out of debt and could afford some comforts they had never had before. The medical picture was troublesome, however. Since the operation 15 months before, she had had an intermittently draining sinus over the left abdominal scar as well as a perineal abscess. The perineal infection subsided, but a year later the patient again developed a perineal abscess. A combined abdominoperineal exploration was made a month later, with the excision of the perineal sinus that communicated with a pelvic abscess; a revision of the ileostomy was also carried out. The patient had a stormy convalescence, and the healing of the abdominal wounds and the perineal wounds was slow.

Despite her discouragement, she no longer became depressed. Her ability to carry on a fairly normal life over the past few years had changed her outlook and attitude, and she survived the postoperative difficulties surprisingly well.

After some years, the patient and her family moved to another part of the country, and she responded to a follow-up questionnaire as follows:

1. She reported her health as fair. She had visited the emergency service of the local hospital for an obstruction of her stoma. A report from the hospital, however, indicated that there had been spontaneous relief of the obstruction. She had a postoperative hernia that interfered with her daily chores; she tired easily; and she was not well enough to seek gainful work.
2. Concerning her depressions, she noted that they recurred at times but that she overcame them with little difficulty. She believed that her depressions were caused by financial troubles and by her husband's and son's ill health. On the whole she remained hopeful. Overt depression was no longer a striking part of the picture.
3. Her ability to show anger, she stated, had improved since psychotherapy. Angry outbursts only lasted a few moments, and she "felt better afterward." She felt more independent and self-assured. (There was no evidence of any paranoid trends or ideas.)
4. She remarked that seeing the psychiatrist had started her on the road to recovery. She had learned to accept her condition and seemed able to take disappointments without collapsing into helpless dependence.

Psychotherapy had not materially helped to reverse the gradual spread of the disease or ward off its complications. Most of the colon disease had been existent before she entered psychotherapy. With this treatment, she was sustained through difficult experiences and was ultimately able to break her infantile dependence upon her mother. Hysterical conversion reactions no longer occurred. Psychotherapy prepared her to accept the frightening "mutilation" of surgery that undoubtedly prolonged her life. But most of all, it helped her to salvage genuine rewards from her life that would otherwise have been denied her.

SUMMARY

There is no question that her earlier intensive psychotherapy had helped her to postpone a colectomy for nearly 20 years. During that time, she was able to establish her own home, to achieve a sense of worth and independence, to make herself less vulnerable to her destructively interfering mother and to establish a firm relationship with her husband and son, whom *she* could support and help.

The patient had desperately needed someone to cling to, and she was able to forge a close bond with her husband in spite of, or perhaps because of, his limited intelligence and lack of education. She was disappointed in her son because of his intellectual deficits and his epilepsy but included him in the tight family unit she created.

How was this patient with so many severe physical illnesses able to carry on without a severe mental breakdown? Reference has already been made to the part played by the family unit that she forged with her husband and son. Additional aids were her relationship to the psychiatrist, her earlier intensive psychotherapy and the timely assistance of the Social Service Department of the hospital.

Experience has shown that the continued support of a physician for indefinite periods of time can play a crucial role in sustaining the ulcerative colitis patient. This was undoubtedly so for this patient, even though later contact was only occasional.

One must recognize, finally, that the character of the therapist was one of the most important elements in the patient's survival. He was unfailingly available, always patient and hopeful and never demanded more than she could sustain. No one who knew her could doubt that his intervention had saved her and her immediate family.

Case Four: A Psychotherapeutic "Failure"

The patient, a 30-year-old man, was a married high school teacher. His first episode of ulcerative colitis had occurred three years before psychotherapy was begun.

The illness started six months after the patient's marriage. He recalled being bitterly disappointed with his wife. Before their marriage he had considered her understanding, mature and cheerful, but afterward he found her moody, demanding, unsupportive and prone to anxiety. She was sexually passive and inhibited, and he angrily described her as "frigid." Nevertheless, although he could intellectualize about their sexual difficulties as "her problem," he acknowledged that he felt sexually inadequate. In a characteristic effort to theorize, he thought that the core of his problem, and probably of his ulcerative colitis, was his need to believe that his wife was "aways right and omnipotent." Whenever he felt guilty for opposing her or felt inadequate, he had an intense need for her reassurance and her repeated statements of approval. Until that need was gratified, his more or less constant but mild diarrhea would become more severe.

The patient came from a devoutly religious family. He was the second of five brothers. His father was a quiet and withdrawn man, occasionally slightly sentimental but lacking genuine compassion for others, according to his son. He was an unsuccessful businessman who relied heavily upon his wife's judgment. His mother was a strong matriarchal figure who controlled her husband and her sons by nagging and by setting high standards that no one seemed able to meet to her satisfaction. She was active in the community and was always ready to give advice and help to those less fortunate than herself. The patient speculated that she was altruistic out of guilt and asserted that he was like his mother in this regard.

According to the patient, he had been a passive, submissive and shy boy until the age of 19, when he suddenly became a socially active rebel. This alteration of his personality proved to be a temporary one, lasting only through his service in the armed forces. When he returned home, his passive dependence on his mother was resumed.

He summed up his conflict a few years after his marriage as coming from "frustrated dependency needs" that he thought had led to his developing colitis shortly afterward.

This patient underwent two periods of psychotherapy, with different male therapists. The first course lasted five months, during which he had 30 treatment sessions. He began this first phase of therapy with the announcement that his wife was pregnant and that he was angry and depressed.

The first therapist was a passive man who had some difficulty coping with his own hostility, from which he retreated into a somewhat aloof, though gentle, posture. He tended to interpret the unconscious conflicts in the patient that concerned his fear of showing anger and of acting more independently. The result of these interpretations was that the patient was confronted almost immediately with a poorer self-image. This confirmed his own view that he was a failure as a man, like his father.

Very early in this first therapy, the patient complained that his doctor was not active enough. He wanted more participation, more "focus." He felt that the therapist should free him from his "irrational" feelings of angry disappointment with his wife and his family for their frequent lack of emotional response.

His early dreams revealed how angrily competitive he was with his elder brother and with his father because of the special interest and attention shown them by his mother. Before his wife left him for two weeks to visit her parents, he dreamed repeatedly of nursing at her breast. His diarrhea promptly intensified, and brooding resentment at feeling "deserted" took over. He now began to quarrel with his mother and his superior at work. Shortly after his wife's departure, he dreamed of solving a difficult family problem for one of his students, after which he felt "warm and accepting." He awoke with intense diarrhea. The therapist kept interpreting everything in terms of the patient's rage at not being treated like a favored child, and the patient's bitter depression deepened. He began to attack his mother and to side with his father. Acting upon his therapist's apparent suggestion to stand on his own feet seemed only to intensify the colitis. By the time his wife returned, he was quite ill, although he managed to keep working. To make matters worse, the patient was told that his therapist would have to leave the clinic and that he would be transferred to another therapist as soon as one was available. The patient swallowed any anger that he felt and said only that he didn't "like it but it can't be helped." He promptly had a dream in which he was a helpless baby being nursed; the breast, however, suddenly became a penis. When he awoke, he was frightened that this meant he might become a homosexual. The therapist stopped the therapy after three weeks, during which the patient talked only of his wife's withdrawal from him and of the baby she would give birth to in three months. He feared that he then would have even less of his wife's attention than before. There was no change in his colitis.

Another therapist was not available for two months, during which the patient managed as best he could. The colitis continued with little improvement.

The second therapy lasted nine months and involved 45 therapeutic interviews. He opened the treatment with an outburst of anger at his first therapist because the latter had been so impassive and neutral. His new therapist proved to be more active, and he "mixed it up" more with his patient. Although he identified them in the same way as the first therapist, he made no attempt to interpret the patient's unconscious conflicts inherited from childhood. He chose to deal with the patient's feelings and responses to his current situation. The content of the therapeutic sessions changed. Now the patient spoke of ongoing conflicts between his wife and his mother and of the helplessness they evoked in him. He recalled his mother's suggestion that he became ill often because marriage demanded an active sexual life. His depression frequently came and went; he quarreled with his brother; he complained about his mother, his father and his present therapist; and he talked hopelessly about not wanting to get well.

He would respond with anger when his competitiveness was pointed out by his therapist. The real problem in this phase of his treatment, as in the first, was that *any* therapy inevitably threatened him initially with having to renounce his yearning to remain attached to a strong care-giving mother or mother surrogate. Perhaps if treatment could have been maintained over several years, the patient might have been gradually weaned. That proved impossible, because the patient suddenly announced that he was leaving the locale for another state, where he had obtained a better position. He discontinued psychotherapy without having achieved substantial symptomatic or somatic improvement.

The personalities of the patient's therapists helped determine the kinds of intervention they used. The first was rather inactive and took a more "analytic" stance in the sense that he was nonresponsive to every assertion of the patient and encouraged his free association of ideas and his finding answers for himself. He occasionally interpreted the destructive aims of the patient's rage; by so doing, he seemed to accentuate the patient's weakness and lack of "masculine" assertiveness. In consequence, this therapist intensified the patient's conflict between his image of himself as helpless and ineffectual and his grandiose ideal of being totally independent and in command of all relationships. All that resulted from this first therapeutic experience were greater self-contempt in the patient for his exposed failings and anger toward the therapist.

The second therapist was more active, made suggestions and encouraged the patient to assume a tough aggressive posture toward the women upon whom he had previously depended. He changed the patient's view of his mother as a victim of an incompetent husband, and he exposed her control of the patient and his father. The result was an effort by the patient to establish guilt-free independence from coercive women. Later, the patient tried to make a dramatic change in his environment, from a protected one to one in which he had a better chance to obtain power legitimately and to become an authority in his own right. No less important was his wish to force a separation from his mother by physically distancing himself from her.

Unfortunately, his psychotherapy was interrupted before he had effectively changed his tendency to identify with powerful women, who still succeeded in arousing his guilt if he dared challenge them. When that happened, he regressed to acting like a dependent child and would become incapable of direct assertion. His depression deepened at the same time, and his diarrhea served as a substitute for the expression of defiance and anger.

Eight years after his treatment was terminated, a long follow-up report was obtained from his attending internist. His physical status had apparently improved moderately, although his disease flared up periodically. He had become successful in his work and exercised more authority at home. The marriage was no more gratifying, but he and his wife now had four children.

The patient ascribed his changed social behavior and his improved effectiveness to his second psychotherapist, whom he recalled with some warmth. Physically, however, the disease process seemed unaffected by psychotherapy or, for that matter, by his medical treatment of diet and steroids.

This patient was apparently not suited for very brief psychotherapy. Whether a long period of treatment would have accomplished more, one cannot say. It seems most unlikely that this man's borderline psychopathological disorder could have been reversed by anything but years of therapy. A sustained relationship with his therapist might have reduced the severity of his recurring attacks of colitis—an effect of long-term therapy that we have observed frequently.

Case Five: A Psychotherapeutic Transference "Cure"

This case illustrates the possibilities for rapid and lasting improvement by a sharply focused uncovering of previously repressed emotional conflicts. The favorable outcome was primarily due to the positive trust in the therapist and to his correctly timed and correctly phrased clarifying interpretations.

The patient was a 22-year-old married woman who was first seen by her therapist in the hospital ward. She had been hospitalized for severe erythema nodosum and moderately severe ulcerative colitis. She was an attractive, quiet and somewhat inhibited young woman who quickly established a friendly, if limited, relationship with her therapist. She was guarded but not hostile or overtly suspicious. She clearly evoked the sympathy of her therapist, who found her thoroughly likable. Nevertheless, after a few visits her therapist realized that beneath her agreeable and compliant exterior lay controlled but intense resentment, stubborn opposition and unverbalized feelings of bitter hostility toward demanding figures of authority.

The patient's symptoms had begun five years earlier with mild diarrhea accompanied by severe erythema nodosum and joint pains. Two months before her hospitalization, she had suffered a severe bout of ulcerative colitis, with a 25-pound weight loss, pain and bloody diarrhea. She also had fever, joint pain and lesions typical of erythema nodosum. She was to remain in the hospital nine weeks. Her psychotherapy was carried out in the ward once weekly for four weeks, until her discharge. It was then continued on an out-patient basis, first weekly, then monthly, over 14 months. The therapy involved 25 sessions altogether.

The patient was married and had one child. She had been actively trying to help her husband set up an independent business while struggling to be available also to her three-year-old son. Her parents were alive but ailing. The mother's problems apparently concerned the patient more than the father's.

She could report no obvious precipitative events prior to her illness.

Despite some early hints of negative feelings toward her father, she claimed that her relations with both parents were comfortable and pleasant. She admitted, however, that as the youngest of several siblings, she had always felt that she was slighted and was treated as the least important member of the family. Because a constant fear in her childhood was that of disappointing her father, she sought to be ingratiatingly obedient. Her attitude toward the mother was a mixture of close dependence and annoyance at her rigidity.

The patient was apparently deeply in love with her husband. She socialized freely and made friends easily. She denied any sexual problems, although she did not always achieve orgasm.

The history of her childhood and of her early adulthood was unusually sparse, and her responses to questions were not so much evasive as empty. She literally seemed to remember little. Her life had apparently consisted of a dull repetition of limited conscious emotional experiences, in which school achievement, financial security and positive recognition by others were her principal goals. She was generally competent but seldom lived up to her own expectations. Like so many repressed people, she filled the self-made gaps in recollection by repeating the usual clichés that everything had been "fine" or that she "had had no problems." The therapist believed that her empty platitudes signified her preoccupation with being considered "normal," "mentally healthy" and acceptable to all. He therefore made the goal of therapy her discovery of the unmistakable connections between her physical symptoms and her emotional reactions to everyday experiences. Not surprisingly, at first she was acutely uncomfortable about having to follow the train of her thoughts and to report them to the therapist. After a brief period of passive waiting, the patient's increasing tension compelled the therapist to express his sympathetic recognition of her embarrassment at opening herself up to him; he also posed open-ended questions designed to uncover her covert feelings about current experiences with significant persons. At first, she applied this "training" in self-examination to defining her attitudes toward hospital personnel, fellow patients and visitors. The inquiry aroused her interest, and quite spontaneously she began to apply the new self-revelation to her feelings about her parents, siblings, husband and child.

As is typical in most patients, the issues involved were ordinary events common to all of us, but which in her case stimulated painful conflicts between her needs for dependency and her secret fantasies of being recognized as special. After a few meetings, once this basic conflict had become evident, she readily admitted that she was bitterly self-critical and often depressed when she failed to obtain admiration and approval, especially from her mother and her father. During her marriage she had grown deeply resentful, because her mother-in-law had failed to show even the limited love and attention that she had enjoyed from her own mother.

Five years earlier, shortly before the onset of her present illness, her father had suffered a severe depression for which he finally had to be hospitalized. Very early in her therapy, after confiding the story, with the aid of the therapist's encouraging tolerance she began to voice her resentment and her hostility toward her father as well as toward her husband. The father, a withdrawn and frequently depressed man, had always been self-absorbed and had ignored her; her husband in the past several months had become too concerned with his work and "took her for granted." A dream immediately afterward of a quarrel with her mother-in-law helped her to realize that she blamed the older woman for her husband's neglect. She reported feeling "very good" after verbalizing her anger at the father, husband and mother-in-law, and she noted with pleasant surprise that her diarrhea had subsided and that her erythematous lesions had become less painful.

In succeeding sessions, she tackled one problem at a time with obvious enthusiasm. First, she admitted guilty fears of ending up with a "nervous breakdown" like her father. Next, she was reassured by the therapist that she was in no danger of developing a psychosis and that her fears were the result of her guilt about her anger toward the father. Once she was able to accept that resentment as natural, she lost the fear of becoming mentally ill. She then worked over her irritation with her husband, which she had again hidden out of guilt. As she grew more self-confident that her need for more interest and attention (which the therapist was obviously providing) was just, the patient expressed more positive feelings about herself. The therapist during these first few weeks was supportive and uncritical; he encouraged her self-discovery by his tacit approval; and he interpreted only superficially the patient's irrational fears of receiving a dreadful punishment for her hostility toward those she loved and depended upon. She frankly admitted that in the case of her mother and her husband, she deeply resented being second in importance. Her husband should have reprimanded his mother for her coldness to his wife. She could now feel less guilt about her father and her wish to stay away from him during his mental illness. In the seventh session, after having been discharged from the hospital free of symptoms, she began to speak hesitantly of her hostility and her critical feelings toward her mother, especially for her lack of sensitivity to the father's illness. Admittedly, the patient had herself taken on some of her mother's negative attitudes, and she regretted having done so. Following this self-confrontation and the verbal attack upon her mother, with whom she clearly identified, the patient developed mild diarrhea. When the therapist suggested that there was a connection between the symptoms and her guilt for harboring critical thoughts about her mother, the diarrhea ended within a day.

The patient was so struck by this evidence of the relationship between feelings and symptoms that she raised the issue of her attitude toward the therapist in the next session. Reluctantly, she admitted her pleasure at seeing him and talking to him, but she confessed that her growing attachment to him increased her anxiety about future sessions. The "confession" of "bad thoughts" was again followed shortly by a return of diarrhea, with morning vomiting. During the next few meetings, her erotic fantasies about her therapist were frankly discussed, including the fantasy in which she shamefacedly associated her "morning sickness" with having a child by him. The therapist made no attempt to pursue these fantasies to their origins in her early childhood wishes for a special closeness to her father. He succeeded in "decompressing" her anxious tension by accepting her wish for an affectionate tie to him as a natural reaction to his interest and availability and to her dependence upon him. The explanation was a partial one, although it was true enough as far as it went. It apparently succeeded in relieving her anxiety, and in place of the desire for closer ties, it encouraged a degree of identification with the therapist, who provided a model of strength and consistency. She remained symptom-free the next eight months of therapy, during which the sessions were reduced by mutual agreement to once every three or four weeks.

In the twentieth meeting, which fell almost exactly on the anniversary of the first session, the patient strongly expressed her negative feelings about having to care for her mother, who now lived in her home. The father remained hospitalized most of the time. With this minor outburst, she suffered a mild attack of erythema nodosum and diarrhea. Both symptoms subsided within a week. The therapist accepted her reactions without comment. Three months later, again by mutual agreement, the therapy was ended. When able to leave the hospital, her father was to be cared for by his sisters. She was still resentful at his total self-absorption. Her mother now lived with her permanently. She ended therapy with a positive statement of her new sense of competence and of her freedom from guilt about hostile thoughts.

Ten years later, she was interviewed for follow-up purposes by another psychiatrist. There had been no further attacks of ulcerative colitis and only rare, minor flare-ups of the erythema nodosum. The patient had two children, felt her marriage to be much more secure and was in fact now pregnant a third time. Her husband's business had prospered with her active help.

She felt that her psychotherapy had been the "main factor" in her recovery. She stated that she had a general feeling of well-being and increased self-confidence. Her improvement had been maintained through a number of severe emotional crises, including the assumption of full responsibility for caring for her psychotically depressed father during his terminal illness.

A summary of the factors in her recovery underscores the positive character traits of the patient that she had brought to treatment. She was bright, in touch with her positive feelings to an extent that is uncommon in severe cases of ulcerative colitis, capable, and strongly motivated toward self-examination. She was able to form a positive working alliance with her therapist that supported her strong hope for recovery. That therapeutic relationship stimulated her suggestibility and her responsiveness to the interpretive and permissive comments of the therapist. Another positive factor in her prognosis was that she had begun treatment before her colon had suffered severe irreversible structural damage. From the viewpoint of her capability to form relationships, she was a relatively individuated woman who could concern herself with others' needs despite her own neurotic conflicts about dependency and guilt for aggressive impulses. Her fear of ending up like her psychotic father proved easy to overcome. Finally, she forged a lasting identification with her therapist, whom she saw as a model of independence who cared for those in need. That identification succeeded also in freeing her from the stringent self-criticism of her conscience for minor "transgressions," such as the fantasy of hostility toward her mother and that of "improper" erotic thoughts about an idealized therapist.

The therapist's technique was a mixture of the cathartic release of impounded feelings, support, and clarifying interpretations of the connections between the patient's guilt and her physical symptoms. He was fairly active with the patient and consistently demonstrated his high interest, empathy and optimism about her recovery.

This was the kind of treatment that might well have been conducted by an informed internist who understood the role of emotional conflicts in predisposing the patient to ulcerative colitis. One of the problems that we have encountered in having internists assume a psychotherapeutic responsibility is their own anxiety about dealing with the patients' anxieties and regressive fantasies about being taken care of. Perhaps periodic consultations with a psychiatrist during the internist's therapeutic efforts would ease that burden. Since the internist is usually the first to meet the patient and to gain his or her trust, it would be a pity if he did not also learn how to deal with the more immediate psychological issues in the patient's illness. More severe sequelae might well be avoided with earlier preventive interventions by the physicians who first treat the ulcerative colitis. The patient described here is an example of an individual who could have been psychotherapeutically treated by the internist at the start of the disease to great advantage.

Chapter Seven

PHYSIOLOGICAL AND PSYCHOLOGICAL RESPONSE TO REMOVAL OF THE COLON

Some physicians feel that surgery should be considered for patients who have suffered with chronic ulcerative colitis more than 10 years, because of the possibility of malignancy developing in the large intestine. This is particularly true for those suffering from long-term pseudopolyposis. It is interesting that in a series of 104 cases, in which the average patient was followed 15 years, not a single patient developed carcinoma of the colon.

One of the most difficult situations is the patient who has frequent hospitalizations and is dependent in his social and business life on the close presence of a toilet. One of our patients, a brilliant student, was able to complete only two years of college credit in a five-year period. He was hospitalized at least two or three times a year and missed classes frequently because of intestinal upsets. There were marked fibrosis and ulceration of the colon. When one of the internists charted a monthly record of the previous five years of the patient's life, it was striking to see how nonproductive the student had been. Surgery was decided upon as the treatment of choice. The following year, he won a scholarship and went on to attain a postgraduate degree in English. Although physically well, he returned four years later for psychotherapy.

The decision to employ surgery rests on any of three factors: (1) It is a necessary and life-saving procedure; (2) the disease process is severely chronic; and (3) the patient has a marked inability to function in important areas.

The operation of choice in our experience is a total colectomy. At our institution, it is extremely rare to leave the rectum in place. An ileostomy may be performed on the patient who is not too ill, followed five to six weeks later by a single-stage total colectomy. Another approach is to perform an ileostomy and upper colectomy as a first stage and a combined abdominoperineal resection as a second stage.

POSTOPERATIVE PROBLEMS

To prevent their becoming discouraged if the situation should arise, patients should be informed before leaving the hospital that they may be required to return for revision of the stoma. In our series of patients, 41 per cent required revision of the stoma.

Only when the patient feels in relative control of his bowel function, and accidents have been virtually eliminated, can a measure of peace of mind be achieved. For many individuals, knowledge offers the best form of control—knowledge of what one can expect prior to surgery, as well as knowledge of how best to care for the skin, eliminate odor and maintain a proper diet once surgery has been performed.

All patients who participated in the "ostomy" clubs indicated that these organizations were a positive force in their early adjustment to ileostomy. The active members are, for the most part, those who have made satisfactory adjustments to their surgery. In addition to providing practical guidance from firsthand experience, they serve as successful figures with whom the patient with a new stoma can positively identify.

Sexual impotence or genital anesthesia is an uncommon consequence of colectomy for ulcerative colitis. Erection results from stimuli traveling along parasympathetic pathways originating in the spinal cord. These nerves originate in the second, third, and fourth sacral segments. The parasympathetic nervi erigentes pass through the inferior hypogastric plexus to supply the pelvic viscera. The fibers are in close proximity to the lateral and anterior walls of the rectum. If they are sectioned during surgery, erectile capacity will be abolished.

Ejaculation is dependent upon the integrity of the sympathetic supply to the internal genitalia. These fibers too are vulnerable during rectal surgery at the sacral promontory. Surgery should be performed as close to the rectal wall as possible to keep nerve damage to a minimum.

Anatomic defects may play a role in a given individual's sexual impotence or genital anesthesia. Just as important are his concept of bodily worth and bodily integrity after surgery and especially the actual and imagined responses of the sexual partner. Our findings support those authors who stress the role of the spouse in later sexual adjustments. The value of a man as a worker or of a woman as an attractive wife is often confirmed through the eyes of the partner. These issues are of particular importance in the colitis population, since the patients are often quite young when colectomy is performed and are at an age when sexual issues are important not only directly but also indirectly, in terms of dating, courting and childbearing.

Fears of inadequacy on the job that disturb some male patients may result from their fear of sexual inadequacy and from excessive concerns about "straining" themselves and injuring the stoma. What one advises the patient about how much to tell his fellow workers and his employers can also be most helpful.

The central role of the surgeon cannot be minimized. It is to him that the patient will usually turn for *all* aspects of his care after a colectomy, not just for surgical adjustments. The patient's dependence upon the internist prior to surgery may now be shifted to the surgeon. Neurotic elements as well as the results of surgery may determine whether the patient will regard the surgeon as healer, omniscient guide and counselor, or as violator and mutilator. The surgeon should be aware of the many emotional difficulties the patient may have in spite of good overall physical functioning. Patients are often reticent about discussing matters concerning bowel function and other intimate problems; unless specifically asked, they may not verbalize their anxieties. It is doubtful that problems will be "suggested" to patients who do not already have them.

Our study group has been interested in the effect of the operative procedure on the patients' psychological health. We were interested in their reaction to the loss of a vital organ and to the resultant changes in their body image. We attempted to differentiate the realistic difficulties that all patients must face following surgery from those that are peculiar to a given individual owing to his or her own personality structure and development. The answers to these studies provide an increased understanding of patient attitudes and of physician attitudes toward this common and major type of surgery.

Although ileostomies have been performed with increasing frequency (it has been estimated that perhaps 20,000 people in the United States have had ileostomies, with more than 5000 persons undergoing this procedure every year), most of the literature to date has been concerned with the surgical and mechanical aspects of managing the stoma, the diet, the appliance and local skin reactions.

It is significant to note that the *emotional* consequences of colectomy have usually been ignored. Many psychiatrists and internists, on the other hand, hestitate to recommend the procedure to patients with ulcerative colitis; they, as well as the patient, often regard it as a mutilation.

Lenneberg et al., in a research and demonstration project prepared by the Office of Vocational Rehabilitation, reported the responses to a questionnaire sent to 1425 persons who had had an ileostomy.[1] A major finding was the state of overall physical well-being. Of these ileostomy patients, 81 per cent described their health as excellent or good. Almost half these patients had been seriously ill chronic invalids for more than five years prior to colectomy. Recovery from surgery was achieved in less than a year by 85 per cent of the patients.

The same study involved interviews with 14 men and 13 women who had had ileostomies. The authors' conclusion was that, although major difficulties in adaptation were rare, a generalized lack of "peace of mind" was common. The good outcomes noted at the functional level were rarely duplicated in terms of the individual's sense of well-being. Of the 14 men, 13 were working full-time. Yet only three of them functioned well psychologically, and at least 10 were using obvious pathogenic defense mechanisms against the painful emotions caused by their ileostomies. For a number of the men, the stoma and its care were a source of resentment. Of the 13 women, 12 were in good health, and all were occupied full-time, either as housewives, students or employees of a business. It appeared that the women functioned at a better level psychologically and were able to accept help for their personal problems far more readily than the men.

As mentioned previously, sexual adequacy following a colectomy preoccupied many patients. In 1958, Stahlgren and Ferguson reported on 62 patients who had had abdominoperineal resections for chronic ulcerative colitis.[2] Of 25 men, 5 had poorer sexual function, 18 showed no impairment and 2 improved their sexual functioning. Of 26 women studied, 2 were worse, 23 showed no impairment and 1 was improved. The authors discussed the importance of the surgical technique involved and decided that surgery for ulcerative colitis could be anatomically more limited and, hence, less damaging than the abdominoperineal resection for cancer. In 1952, Sutherland et al. described the sexual performance of male patients who had had colostomies for cancer.[3] Of 29 men, 14 were totally impotent, 5 had decreased erectile strength and only 7 were unimpaired. In 1965, a questionnaire sent to 10 surgeons in the United States showed that the incidence of sexual impotence following abdominoperineal resection for cancer of the rectum varied from 53 per cent to 100 per cent, with an average incidence of 76 per cent.[4]

Various authors recognize the vital impact of the spouse and the family on the colectomy patient. Dyk and Sutherland reported in 1956 on the reactions of the spouse and other family members to the patient with a colostomy.[5] They described some of the difficulties that followed the procedure. The men relied on their wives to be nurses during the immediate postoperative period, while women preferred other women to provide this kind of help. The husband's perception of his wife as a person who could accept the sight and smell of his wound and stoma in the immediate postoperative stage was most important. The authors noted that the wives often disparaged their sick husbands, at times quite openly. They felt that he now had diminished value because his social activities and his income were reduced and because he was a possible source of embarrassment to them. They believed their husbands' bodies were more fragile and that the stoma was ugly.

The male spouse, on the other hand, tended to be more supportive of his wife and less disturbed by the stoma. Nevertheless, women had a greater fear than men of not being physically acceptable to their spouses.

The authors stated that the marital relationship of any colostomy patient was a "powerful force for good or evil," and the spouse was often the key to the patient's eventual success or failure in adapting to his disability.

Lenneberg et al. state that family members require professional attention for their own sakes as well as for the patient, since family acceptance can be the most important influence on the patient's future adaptation.

Concerning ultimate physical adjustment to the appliance itself, Lenneberg et al. report that 40 per cent of respondents indicated that they had appliance problems: Fifty-four per cent had skin trouble, and 46 per cent had problems with odor. Their conclusion is that the influence of appliance failures on the rehabilitation of the ileostomy patient is profound. The patients described severe humiliation at any spillage or accident, at times to the point of considering suicide. Many were phobic concerning the noise of gas or its odor. Some had a pathological fear of injuring the stoma that interfered with their ability to pursue employment. It was not uncommon for patients to develop rituals as a method of regaining a sense of control. Some became food faddists in an effort to regulate input when bowel control had been lost.

Small reported two case studies of individuals with stomas whom he treated psychotherapeutically.[6] In this setting, he was able to explore the alterations in body image and the fantasies engendered by the creation of an artificial organ of elimination.

A Manual for Ileostomy Clubs describes the ileostomy and colostomy mutual aid groups and their role in the adjustment of these patients, both before and after surgery.[7] These groups are now more than 20 years old and exist in many cities throughout the United States and abroad. Their work is accomplished during meetings, regular social gatherings and visits to pre- and postoperative patients; their most important function is to test new prosthetic equipment as it becomes available.

A group of 41 patients with chronic ulcerative colitis who ultimately underwent surgery was studied at The Columbia–Presbyterian Medical Center, New York, by a team including two psychiatrists and a surgeon.[8,9] The patients were asked to respond to a questionnaire that covered the presurgical period, the immediate postsurgical period and the overall long-term adjustment since surgery.

All except one patient indicated that their general health was excellent or "very good." Most felt that having an ileostomy was preferable to living with severe ulcerative colitis. One patient put it this way: "Ileostomy was the best thing that has ever happened to me and I'm glad I no longer have to live in the bathroom." Another patient said that "ileostomy means freedom" and that life had expanded for her following surgery.

In general, however, they felt that they had received little real preparation for surgery; many felt shock on first looking at the stoma. Others said that the surgeons and the nurses were unable to instruct them in the day-to-day management of the appliance. Many volunteered that the person most helpful to them was a member of the local ileostomy club. Patients who were visited after surgery indicated that visits prior to surgery also would have been even more helpful.

The most important issues were the personal and interpersonal ones. Patients invariably saw the ileostomy in relationship to key figures in their lives. One woman stated that she was reassured following surgery that her husband did not seem to mind her stoma and that "he didn't care which end I went to the bathroom from." A male patient said that he was helped most by the supportive attitude of his superiors and his co-workers on the job. Most had great difficulty in explaining the operation and its attendant problems to friends; one person said that she did not disclose that she had had an ileostomy to anyone but had kept the matter completely private. Several were concerned that acquaintances would react with horror or disgust. They frequently ascribed their sexual performance problems to anticipating this same reaction from their partners.

Many knew they had emotional problems before and after colectomy, while others denied serious emotional difficulties. Five patients who disclaimed any history of emotional problems had had more than two years of psychotherapy. One was an in-patient at the New York State Psychiatric Institute, and one had not attended school for four years because of multiple phobias, including the fear of losing bowel control.

A variety of attitudes toward psychiatry were expressed by these patients. One patient felt that any emotional disorders were a result of the disease process itself and that good adjustment was due to "will and fight." Another who had had psychotherapy felt that "it was of no help whatsoever" and that "emotional factors are unimportant." One said that psychiatry had led to a cure for many of his problems, but he was "still stuck with an ileostomy." Others felt that if they had had psychiatric treatment at an earlier stage, they would not have needed the ileostomy at all; one emphasized that a psychiatrist should have been available during the complete period of hospitalization for surgery.

The initial reaction to surgery of virtually all ileostomy patients was depression. As psychological test data suggest, even patients with a facade of good spirits were often depressed, and for many reasons.[10] First, there was the loss of a highly valued organ; depression is an expected reaction to significant loss. An additional component of the depressed state is the sense of having been mutilated. No matter how well instructed they were prior to surgery, the patients reacted to their first sight of the colostomy itself with shock. Men regarded this surgery at times as a castration; some unconsciously perceived the initial bleeding from the stoma as menstruation and hence as evidence of feminization. Women were concerned that they had been violated and eviscerated. Both sexes felt that their bodies had been made weaker, more fragile and unattractive, and they thought that they were now inferior. Each patient blamed the mutilation on himself, because he was too dependent on the surgeon at this time to allow any feelings of anger to emerge. This *impounding of resentment* further contributes to depression.

Added to the sense of loss and of mutilation is the inescapable situation of being unable to avoid violating the established social *code of cleanliness*. Just as in the past, to soil oneself was to risk the loss of acceptance and love; thus, following surgery, many feared becoming disgusting to others.

Once the initial shock and the consequent depressive state have passed, many patients do well. Their response in the first year or so after surgery would appear to be the crucial determinant in their eventual adaptation. The more successful patients made use of obsessional defenses such as increased cleanliness, tidiness and concern with external appearances. Many used denial, hypomania and counterphobia, which suggested a defense reaction against a feeling of helplessness.[11] Some, particularly the females, became exhibitionistic in terms of both their stoma and their body in general, but these were few in number.

CHANGES IN BODY IMAGE

Because of the limitations of questionnaires, it was felt that more intensive interviews would be useful. Accordingly, from the respondents, four patients with ileal stomas established at least five years were selected for interview.[12] All four had been in psychotherapy: two in analysis and two in dynamic psychotherapy. All four were women 23 to 63 years of age. Because all had been in therapy, this undoubtedly introduced a bias, so these patients may not be representative of the entire group of respondents. They were open in speaking about intimate factors in their lives, however, and gave us permission to consult with the psychoanalyst or the psychotherapist, who provided further data. Nevertheless, the main finding from the lengthy interviews—that despite the seemingly good adjustment to the ileostomy, psychological problems remained—may have more than limited application.

Five significant phenomena were noted in these patients.

1. Phantom Bowel. Many patients stated that, for a few days to two weeks following total colectomy and ileostomy, they had a sense of fullness and a strong urge to defecate from a nonexistent rectum. Patients in our series regularly described this phenomenon. It probably expresses both the persistence of the individual's body image after the loss of an organ and a powerful desire to maintain body integrity, even in fantasy. The phantom bowel occurs during the immediate postoperative period, when the body has undergone a profound change and the ego has not yet begun to cope with and integrate that change.

2. The Stoma as Phallus. Previous discussions in the literature of patients' responses to ileostomy and colostomy have emphasized the experience as a *loss*: the loss of a prized organ, the bowel; the loss of anal sphincter control; and the loss of physical attractiveness. It is not surprising to note that patients who underwent colectomy for carcinoma of the large intestine often responded to these losses with a major depression, and frequently a year or more elapsed before some were able to emerge from it.[9]

Paradoxically, the women in our series reacted to their stoma as if it were a *gain*. One patient had the idea that the stoma looked like a penis that underwent erection during emotional stimulation. It was an organ that she considered disgusting but fascinating. It appeared to have a will of its own. Although embarrassed by her expressed fantasy, she seemed to enjoy the exhibitionism of discussing it.

Another patient was not fully conscious of this identification, but her actions and fantasies betrayed her equation of stoma and phallus. She would react with the coy modesty usually associated with uncovering the genital areas when the stoma was exposed. She felt it made her special and unique, and she frankly did not wish to give it up and to return to her prior anatomical state.

A third patient felt that the stoma was an asset and was proud of it. Her appliance was seen as part of the stoma, incorporating both into one bodily organ. During masturbation, she would consciously fantasize that the long, flexible appliance was a man's penis.

Other workers have also noted the equation of intestinal stoma and phallus. Small described a 36-year-old man who underwent ileostomy after 17 years of ulcerative colitis.[6] Prior to the ileostomy, his direct handling of his genitals for pleasure was inhibited. Following surgery, he freely stimulated the stoma rhythmically during the cleaning process. It would then enlarge and become stiffer—"like when you rub down here," he stated, pointing to his genitals. The nurses were upset because he would stimulate his stoma beyond its hygienic need. Small noted that erogenous zones are typically located where skin and mucous membranes meet, and that this type of junction has special properties that arouse sensation and emotion. Under the unique conditions of ileostomy surgery, a part of the body not previously exposed can apparently become such a surface organ.

3. Exhibitionism. A special example of the equation "stoma equals phallus" is the remarkable exhibitionism of patients with ileostomies. Nurses' notes indicated that one patient openly engaged in sex play with her boyfriend in a ward shortly after surgery. Her first postoperative sexual intercourse was also inappropriately public. All the patients wished to show their equipment; this becomes more understandable when the appliance and other equipment are seen as an extension of the stoma. One patient brought a kit with her to the interview and described the types of glue and powder that were most effective. She also related dreams of taking off the appliance and of showing the stoma to others.

Many patients who are active in ileostomy clubs regularly volunteer to serve as demonstrators during lectures to medical students, nurses and physicians. They seem especially pleased to disrobe for a large, mixed audience. One of the four patients in this series described her satisfaction in teaching medical students about ileostomies.

4. Erotic Transference to Surgeon. One patient was quite open in expressing gratitude to her analyst, who had helped her prepare for the trauma of surgery by working through her anxieties beforehand. Yet it appears that frequently the surgeon becomes even more significant in this type of relationship. A second patient described her surgeon in openly erotic terms, stating that she had a "crush" on him. She felt that he was charismatic and powerful and indicated that she told him things that she did not reveal "to my own analyst."

Another patient felt that her psychiatrist had done little for her following surgery but admitted that she looked forward with excitement to her monthly visits to her surgeon.

A fourth patient agreed to return to participate in her surgeon's research on the intestinal tract because she "loved" being his subject. The relationship was highly eroticized in her mind.

5. Personality, Defense Mechanisms and Life Style. All the patients were busy, energetic women involved in many varied activities. These findings were compatible with those of our first study, which revealed a strikingly high level of social and vocational functioning.

The patients boasted of their prowess and refused to see themselves as crippled or disabled. A dependent or weak self-image was totally abhorrent. On the contrary, they dared to swim in the coldest waters and eat the spiciest foods (against usual medical advice for ileostomy patients). They claimed that they had few problems, and that they could handle those they had. One might have expected them to extract *some* secondary gain from claimed disabilities; none did.

All four women stated that depression was virtually absent, and in fact they appeared mildly hypomanic. During the interviews they were restless, busy and active; there was an aggressive, controlling component to their behavior as well.

In character, they appear to be much like the phallic-narcissistic type originally described by Reich. Reich states that the phallic character occurs infrequently in women but that many productive, energetic women do belong to this group.[11] In the psychoanalysis of this character type, an identification of the total ego with the phallus is observed; in women, the fantasy of having a penis is common. Reich feels that these patients have exhibitionistic tendencies as well.

Denial, hypomania and counterphobic mechanisms were the most prominent defenses in our group of patients and probably protected them from feelings of hopelessness and mutilation.

SUMMARY

Total colectomy is becoming an increasingly common procedure, and the creation of a permanent ileostomy or colostomy should no longer be seen as a necessarily "mutilating" procedure. The physical adaptation to these artificial organs is accomplished more readily, however, than the emotional adaptation. Many patients who function extremely well in social activities, school and work do not evidence the concomitant sense of well-being that one might expect.

Acceptance of the ileostomy by key figures in the patient's life (family, employer, and so forth) is essential to successful adaptation. Visits by local ileostomy club members are very helpful, both in training prospective and new patients and in providing successful models for identification.

Physicians must be aware of the many conscious and unconscious fantasies and the emotional conflicts following surgery that a patient may experience covertly in spite of apparently good overall functioning.

References

1. Lenneberg, E., et al. The Ileostomy Patient. Report of a research and demonstration project, 233. Q. T., Inc., Boston, 1962. Under a grant from the Office of Vocational Rehabilitation.
2. Stahlgren, L. H., and Ferguson, L. K. Influence on sexual function of abdominoperineal resection for ulcerative colitis. N. Engl. J. Med. *259*:873, 1958.
3. Sutherland, A. M., et al. The psychological impact of cancer and cancer surgery. Cancer *5*:857, 1952.
4. Bernstein, W. C. Sexual dysfunction following radical surgery for cancer of rectum and sigmoid colon. Medical Aspects of Human Sexuality, March, 1072, pp. 156–163.
5. Dyk, R. B., and Sutherland, A. M. Adaptation of the spouse and other family members to the colostomy patient. Cancer *9*:123, 1956.
6. Small, S. M. Validation of libido theory. Psychiatr. Q. *27*:38, 1953.
7. Manual for Ileostomy Patients. Issued by Q. T., Inc., Boston, 1964.
8. Druss, R. G., O'Connor, J. F., Prudden, J. F., and Stern, L. O. Psychologic response to colectomy. Arch. Gen. Psychiatry *18*:53, 1968.
9. Druss, R. G., O'Connor, J. F., and Stern, L. O. Psychologic response to colectomy. II. Adjustment to a permanent colostomy. Arch. Gen. Psychiatry *20*:419, 1969.
10. Orbach, C. E., and Tallent, N. Modification of perceived body and of body concepts. Arch. Gen. Psychiatry *12*:126, 1965.
11. Reich, W. Character Analysis. Orgone Institute Press, New York, 1949, p. 202.
12. Druss, R. G., O'Connor, J. F., and Stern, L. O. Changes in body image following ileostomy. Psychoanal. Q. *41*:195, 1972.

Chapter Eight

SUMMARY AND CONCLUSIONS

The definition of the etiological factors in any chronic disease requires an accurate interpretation of the relative contributions of genetic endowment, constitutional vulnerability, intrapsychic processes and the external environment. In some illnesses, heredity is the predominant factor; in others, the disposition to a particular somatic breakdown seems to have been determined largely by the vicissitudes of intrauterine, neonatal and infantile experiences. Still other victims of chronic illness respond with persistent or recurrent somatic dysfunction to psychologically induced conflicts of motivation that are accompanied by prolonged emotional overactivity. A large percentage of colitis sufferers are victims of environmental pathogens and unusual stress combined with one or more of the other factors.

We remain uncertain about the degree and the precise nature of genetic and constitutional vulnerability in the development of chronic ulcerative colitis. Our efforts have been directed primarily at interpreting the complex role of mental processes, motivational conflict and loss of emotional control in the evolution of the disease, as well as determining the responsiveness of colitis to psychotherapy. This study has dealt only with the environment's responsibility for psychological stress upon the patient.

We do not claim that ulcerative colitis is "caused" by unusual reactions of the mind alone; we claim only that these reactions almost always play a vital role in the interaction of the four etiological determinants. In trying to decipher the psychical elements in any illness, one must reckon with their variable significance in a given case. The intrapsychical processes may, for example, predispose to the actual development of the disease; in many cases, however, they may be secondary reactions to the symptoms and to the disability caused by the disease that reinforce and intensify that disability. They may also reflect a combination of causal ingredients, which seems to be the usual situation in chronic ulcerative colitis.

Predisposition to ulcerative colitis originates in mental reactions of a peculiar and specific kind that play a significant part in all patients—and a primary role in some. These predisposing forces are released, we believe, when symbiotic-like attachments to figures of dependency in the victim's past and present life persist. The consequence of such extreme and inappropriate emotional dependence is lasting emotional reactions that involve the body's responses in pathological ways.

Symbiotic-like needs for dependency in any adult are sooner or later doomed to frustration. Angry helplessness follows and may become so intense that depressive apathy may ultimately take over. Statements or acts of aggression by the patient in that state can no longer kindle hopes of future comfort or safety through dependency. In the extreme instance, he or she becomes increasingly withdrawn and distrustful. Direct emotional expression becomes increasingly difficult and is replaced by a nonverbal discharge through activation of an internal organ system. This bodily reaction, which may be compared to that of the infant, cannot, however, express a specific emotional state. It can signify rage, anxious helplessness, a need to suffer or even a suicidal wish to die.

A change in this pathological state may result from the tolerant and unrejecting dependence allowed the patient in therapy. Some ulcerative colitis sufferers, like the analyzed patient in Case One, come to idealize their therapist to the point that their mental image of him as a constant and supportive figure is carried as a magic talisman. If the idealization is to alter their vulnerability and excessive sensitivity to disappointment, they must also be able to *identify* themselves with the idealized therapist's image. Unconsciously, his strengths and his admired traits have been assimilated by these patients, becoming a new addition to their character armor and ways of perceiving reality. Such identifications are most likely to occur in psychoanalytical therapies but can also be seen after less intensive therapies. In both instances, the therapist has, among other things, neutralized the patient's belief in the power of the original object of dependency to hurt him. In its place, the therapist has offered himself as a good and consistent parent surrogate. In patients who undergo lasting positive changes, the symbiotic-like dependency is thus replaced, through the medium of new insight and new identifications, by pleasurable independence, successful individuation and tolerance of separateness in intimacy. At the same time, pathogenic somatic activity becomes less important as a maladaptive mode of emotional discharge.

This describes what we believe to be the source of the psychological predisposition to morbid physical reactions to the stress and demands of everyday life. Given the maldevelopment of faulty emotional factors, other agents—in ways we can only speculate—reduce the structural tolerance of the colon to abnormally intense activation and to functional disruption from psychological excitation. It is then that the target organ becomes vulnerable to tissue breakdown in some individuals. Vascular disturbances in the colon seem to be a major factor in this local tissue destruction and in the faulty healing of the colon that characterizes chronic ulcerative colitis.

Treatment of ulcerative colitis requires the combined efforts of internist, psychiatrist and surgeon. The use of steroids to mitigate acute flare-ups, and the performance of colectomy when severely diseased organs make recovery of function impossible, remain lifesaving procedures. The addition of judiciously selected psychotherapeutic interventions materially improves the chances for lasting improvement and even for total recovery. A proper choice of intervention and a good match between the personality style of the therapist and that of the patient are essential, however, if psychotherapy is to be helpful. There are undoubtedly many cases in which an effective job of psychotherapy could be done by an internist, possibly in occasional consultation with an experienced psychiatrist.

The relationship of ulcerative colitis to granulomatous disease of the colon is not yet clarified. Psychotherapy is not clearly established as a "curative" procedure for granulomatous disease. Nevertheless, many patients are materially helped by psychotherapy in their adjustment to a stubbornly recurring illness. There is also reason to believe that remissions may be prolonged by long-term psychotherapy. Very brief therapy in this group of patients is probably of little lasting value.

The contribution of psychiatry to a fuller understanding and to a more successful treatment of both ulcerative colitis and granulomatous disease of the colon remains controversial in some medical circles. We believe that the stubborn refusal to consider mental etiological factors exposes colitis sufferers to serious and needless risks. It is perhaps the unfortunate result of a tendency of some medical practitioners to treat patients' organs mechanically. As do other humanist physicians, the psychiatrist who works with somatic illness tries to view the patient as a whole and to see his illness as an outcome of many operant pathogenic factors. We can only hope that the work and theories of psychodynamics and of psychotherapy described here will advance that viewpoint. Without sacrificing the important pharmacological and surgical contributions to treatment, a more deliberate and more prolonged use of dynamic psychotherapy can only help the colitis patient and reduce his burden of disability.

INDEX

Page numbers in *italics* refer to illustrations; those followed by t denote tables.